5 Ingredients Smoothie, 5 Exercises,5 Days Results

Detox, Cleanse and Weight Loss Smoothie Recipes Book

< Kate Dowers >

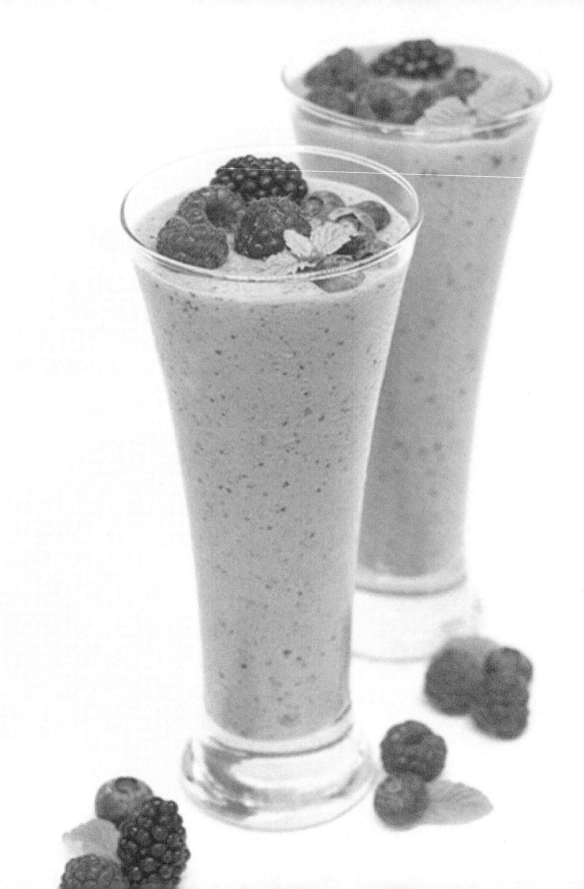

Get our new release for FREE!

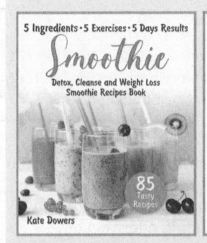

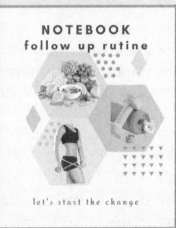

Sing up to our newsletter to get the future release absolutely Free!

https://mailchi.mp/b7abe36ee0fc/kate-dowers

Table of Contents

Green Smoothie Recipes 45

Chapter 4

Tasty Detox Smoothie Recipes 71

Chapter 5

Chapter 6

Introduction

Before we start, I would like you to answer a few questions. How many times have you tried to change your diet to lose weight, or just to adopt a healthier lifestyle? How many times did the plan work? If it didn't, what was the reason? I bet you were able to answer the first two questions but got stuck on the third one. That's normal because many people starting their weight loss (or glow-up) journey blindly follow trends without actually knowing what is good for their body. Everyone is different and so are their bodies. Therefore, what's working for one person might not work for another. One more thing people seem to get stuck on is what food they should consume based on their goals. The result you will achieve depends on the category of foods you consume, and that will look different for each person. For instance, an overweight person trying to lose weight will not have the same nutritional requirements as a fit person who just wants an extra health boost. The differences lie deep down in the details, and to achieve effective results, you have to dig in; that's when this book steps in to help you out.

I want to share my experience with losing weight and how I managed to switch to a better and healthier lifestyle. Being a 35-year-old mother, I can relate to people my age, especially women, who constantly try to reach their fitness goals but somehow keep going back to square one. Let me tell you, I was the same. I was physically tired and stressed out all the time. I wanted to feel better, but I didn't know-how. So I started researching and learning everything I could about health. I learned how factors like nutrition, diet, fitness, and self-care play a crucial role in keeping us healthy and started incorporating little habits into my daily routine. I can proudly say that I am at a point in my life where I am satisfied with my body and my lifestyle. As a nutrition and fitness consultant, I want to pass on those tips and habits that made a big difference for me. This book serves as a starting point for those trying to start a fitness journey. It will help you get a little closer to your goal with each passing day.

This book is carefully curated, keeping in mind the nutrition requirements of each body type and goal. It answers all the questions you might have when starting to get fit and healthy. It is also helpful for those looking to tweak their daily diet with something more nutritious. When I started my journey, the one change in my lifestyle that helped the most was introducing smoothies. You cannot imagine how a smoothie with, or in place of a meal (preferably breakfast), does wonders for your skin and body. A glass full of blended fruits, vegetables, and other nutrient-dense foods is the perfect way to start the day. It keeps you feeling full for a long time and detoxifies your body. The best part is that if you don't like the taste of an ingredient, you can change it! Add in some of your favorite fruits, seeds, nuts, or whatever else you want, and easily make it your kind of smoothie! Smoothies are so versatile—some contain only vegetables, some only fruits, and nuts, and sometimes it's a mix of everything. It depends on your fitness goals and, of course, your tastes. Don't have enough ingredients? Don't worry, this book includes tons of smoothie recipes you can make with as few as five ingredients! Combine this smoothie diet with daily exercises, and you will reach your goals much faster. Combining exercise with a healthy diet not only improves your physical health but also keeps you mentally fit. Daily exercise increases your metabolism, which helps maintain weight loss and keeps you healthy for a long time. It has been proven that having a nutrition-packed diet and exercising daily results in a lower risk of obesity, heart problems, and other fatal diseases. Exercise, especially when combined with a healthy diet, improves your sleep cycle and reduces stress. The benefits are endless. Achieve easily your diet and healthy lifestyle goals by combining a simple smoothie diet and some easy and basic exercises. Throw in some crunches, planks, and sit-ups along with your smoothie diet and see your body transform! Don't know where you start from – don't worry I prepared for you a 5 days program in the final chapters of the book that you can easily multiply in a larger 20 days program that will consolidate the results and will form power of habit. In no time you will fall in love with this new healthier you.

A quick reminder: No matter how great a diet is, it shouldn't be done excessively. Many people fall for various diet trends and go on crash diets, which don't work. They are short-term, and you will eventually gain that weight back. You don't have to starve yourself or skip meals to get fit. You only need to make some small changes in your daily diet, and you will be good to go. Smoothies can be a meal replacement—but they are also a wonderful addition to your daily meals to improve your health. Replace that packet of Doritos or your evening snack with a delicious smoothie and notice the difference. You will look and feel good.

So, hop on this journey with me and learn some amazing tips and tricks that help weight loss. By the time you reach the end of this book, you will know everything you need to start your fitness journey off on the right foot. At the end of all those delicious smoothie recipes you will find a kick-start 5 days plan that will help you:

·Form a healthy routine that will change your overall well-being,

·Will consolidate habits through which you will stay feet, gain a better sleep, detox your body and increase your energy levels

Along with that, you will get many wholesome smoothie recipes that you can make with just five ingredients! If you utilize the information given in the book, you can start to see results in just five days (yes that's right, just five days), so without further ado, let's dive right in.

Chapter 1
Seven Steps to Make the Perfect Smoothie

Smoothies have become quite popular recently because of the incredible amount of benefits they provide. These versatile drinks can be made using a mix of different fruits and veggies for your early morning breakfast or a post-workout energy booster. They can also be part of your meal, based on the ingredients you add. Even in your busiest hours, you can quickly add fruits and veggies to a blender, and take the smoothie with you. If you don't like drinking the thicker textures, turn your smoothie into a smoothie bowl, It is that easy. However, if you are a beginner, you might get confused about the process. To help you with that, I have broken it down into seven easy steps. These steps involve the basic principles you can follow to make the perfect smoothie blend.

1. **Choose your recipe:** Find your favorite smoothie recipe either from the internet or this book and prepare your ingredients. Make sure you have all the ingredients on hand. If you don't have the same ingredients, you can switch them up with the ones that have a similar texture, or take a trip to the grocery store.

2. **Add your liquid:** You can add plain filtered water, coconut water, or even infused water. You can also add some protein powder at this stage and blend it up a bit to avoid lumping.

3. **Add your base:** You can add milk (plant-based or regular) or juice of your choice. You can also add some yogurt to get a creamier texture or some ice cubes to smoothen the blending process.

4. **Add fruits and/or vegetables:** Throw in the fruits and vegetables you prepared in the first step. Don't forget to wash them!

5. **Optional add-ins:** Now is the time to spice it up. You can add ginger, cinnamon, nuts, turmeric, or any superfood you like. These add-ins to your smoothie will give you a much-needed boost and keep you energized for the whole day. They also make your smoothie thicker, which is perfect if you are a smoothie bowl fan.

6. **Blend:** Blend all the ingredients until you get a smooth texture.

7. **Enjoy** your smoothie!

Quick Tip: Make sure that the amount of ingredients is the same as mentioned in the recipe. Otherwise, your smoothie might not turn out to be as good. Also, if you don't balance out the number of ingredients, you might consume more calories than you expected.

You now have a step-by-step process to make the perfect smoothie. However, even after following all the steps, you still might not get the desired results. Sometimes the solution is too runny, other times it's all lumpy and full of little chunks. So, what to do to get the perfect blend every time? As you know, every smoothie has its basic components such as ingredients, texture, and the tools you use to make your smoothie. It also involves how long you blend the smoothie among other things. Here are some tips and tricks you can use when you are not having the ideal smoothie day.

Tips and Tricks for Making the Perfect Blend
How to Improve the Texture of Your Smoothie
If you think your smoothie is too runny, try adding some frozen fruit to it. You can also add some fiber or protein-like oats, chia, or protein powder to make it thicker. Also, avoid mixing fruits and vegetables that are all juicy or watery. Instead, have a mix of both juicy and fibrous ingredients to get a perfect consistency.

What Part of the Fruit or Vegetable to Add
While making a smoothie, you need to pay attention to what parts of a fruit or vegetable you are adding. For instance, if you add lemon to your smoothie, peel it and remove the seeds; otherwise, your smoothie will be bitter. If you don't have a strong blender, chop up the fruits and vegetables to avoid a grainy smoothie texture.

What Kind of Nuts to Add
Nuts are packed with nutrients including fiber, magnesium, iron, calcium, vitamin E, and healthy fats. You can add any kind of nut to your smoothies to get that extra boost of energy. However, adding nuts in large amounts can have the opposite effect on your diet. So, make sure to limit the amount to one ounce or less to balance the calorie count.

What is the Best Order to Add in Ingredients?

Adding the ingredients in the correct order helps in blending the smoothie to the perfect consistency. Start with adding your liquids. If you want to add some leafy greens to your smoothie, make sure to blend them first to break them down easily. Then add in the rest of your fruits and veggies and blend them up. Last, add your fiber and spices and blend it all until smooth.

The Difference Between Frozen and Fresh Ingredients

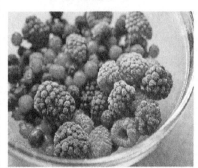 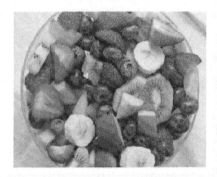

Most people think that fresh ingredients are a healthier and better option. But according to the International Food Information Council, the nutritional value according to the International Food Information Council, the nutritional value content in frozen food is just as high as the fresh food (Winchester Hospital, n.d.). That is because most fruits are picked when they are fresh and ripe and frozen immediately, retaining the nutrients this way. Then they are sent to the stores right after.

Here are some benefits of frozen fruits and vegetables:

●They are cheaper: Frozen foods are cheaper and can be accessed even in off-seasons. They are also available in areas where fresh produce is more difficult to obtain.

●They last longer: You can buy them in bulk and store them in your freezer for a

long time. As fruits don't go through a blanching process, they keep their flavor and nutrients even after a few months.

●Thicker and creamier smoothies: When it comes to making smoothies, frozen fruits are the best choice, especially during summer. Using frozen fruits in your smoothies gives them a creamier and smooth texture. It's almost like you are having a fruity milkshake!

●Time-saving: With frozen fruits, you don't have to cut anything. You can put them directly into the blender and save time. You don't even have to use ice cubes.

If you don't have frozen fruit, freeze your fresh fruit for 30 minutes or overnight before blending, or add about one cup of ice and blend until smooth! Fruits such as bananas, pineapples, mangoes, strawberries, and blueberries make the perfect blend when frozen. So, stack some frozen fruit in your freezer and use them to make creamy and delicious smoothies. The same concept applies to veggies.

Choosing the Right Blender

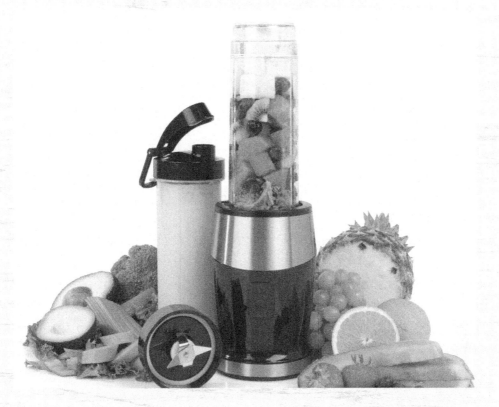

Most blenders out there can make smoothies, but you need to find the one that works best for you. A good blender with durability and high-class performance can raise your smoothie game a notch. Here are the top three recommended blenders based on their speed, immersion, and durability:

1.**Vitamix 5200**

Vitamix is the most popular brand in the world of smoothie blenders. Vitamix 5200 is one of the best editions of blenders from the Vitamix family. It is durable, it is strong, and it has the best market value. It has a patented tamper tool that can blend any ingredient you add to your smoothie, be it fresh or frozen, cut, or uncut. If you are looking to invest in something long-term, this one's for you. Choosing the Right Blender.

2. <u>Nutribullet 600</u>

If you are on a budget and are looking for something more affordable that doesn't take much space in your kitchen, go for this one. It is one of the best single-serve smoothie blenders on the market. It comes with bullet-shaped cups that are perfect for one smoothie and also easier to clean. It is small but powerful, which makes it the perfect addition for people living alone.

3. <u>Blendtec Total Blender</u>

It has a 1500 watt motor, a futuristic electronic display, no knobs or dials, and includes a 96-ounce jar along with a book of over 100 recipes. Blendtec is also a very popular name in the market. This blender comes with a massive 96-ounce jar and is perfect for big families. It has an inbuilt smoothie sensor, which automatically detects when the smoothie is done. You can rest assured that you would get a perfect smoothie texture every time.

The process of blending a perfect smoothie is not that intimidating. You just have to have the right directions and tools, and you can achieve great results every time.

Chapter 2
How Smoothies Can Boost Metabolism by Turning off Fat Genes

Importance of Losing Excess Weight

Why is it important to lose extra weight? Is it just because you want to look good? Sure, that's one of the reasons but not the only reason. Here are five more:

1. Lessen the risk of joint pain: One important reason to lose weight is to prevent your body from developing diseases and joint pain. Overweight people have a higher risk of diseases such as osteoarthritis. Thus, losing weight will lower the risk of joint pains and keep you more active for many years to come.

2. Improved sleep cycle: Losing weight improves your sleep cycle and keeps your metabolic rate in check.

3. Better immune system: When you switch to a healthier diet, you give your body the right nutrients that support muscle growth and a better immune system.

4. Your food will taste better: According to Stanford University researchers, overweight people tend to get dull taste buds over time due to overuse (MacMillan, 2015). So, eating right may help your taste sensitivity and make your food taste better.

Improved memory: Having weak memory can be one of the risks of being overweight. But, avoiding sugar and eating foods good for your body as well as your brain can improve your memory.

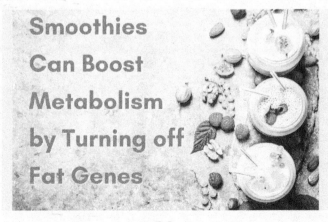

How Smoothies Can Help Weight Loss

Smoothies are the best way to soak up all the essential nutrients you need daily. The blend of different fruits, vegetables, fiber, and fats provides your body with omega-3 fats, vitamins, minerals, antioxidants, and phytochemicals. With the right ingredients, smoothies can improve your metabolism and keep you active for the rest of the day. Improved metabolism helps you burn more calories and lose weight faster. So, if you want to lose weight, then making a smoothie packed with nutrient-dense ingredients is the way to go. The best part about smoothies is the ability to change the ingredients based on your liking and calorie intake needs. The enzymes present in many fruits and vegetables help dissolve fat from your body and regulate your circulatory system. You can customize your smoothie into a low-calorie, nutrition-rich blend that not only improves your metabolic rate but also keeps your blood sugar level in check. Ingredients such as chia seeds, green tea, ginger, cinnamon, and avocados help boost your energy and keep you fuller. Adding spices like turmeric, cayenne pepper, or black pepper help in lessening food cravings and quickening the fat-burning process.

Combining the right fruits, vegetables, and nuts rich in antioxidants, fatty acids, vitamins, and minerals helps support a healthy immune system, which in turn protects your body from diseases. Ingredients like berries, seeds, yogurt, and nuts are rich in vitamins and minerals, nutrients that help build a better immune system. A better immune system contributes to faster weight loss. It keeps your body weight regulated and prevents you from gaining it back.

Another way smoothies help in weight loss is through hydration. As you know, hydration is the key to keeping your weight in check and detoxifying your body. But if you don't like sipping on plain water, try having a smoothie with a large amount of water-rich fruits and vegetables. Hydrating your body keeps your body process working smoothly, which increases your metabolic rate and helps you shred that extra fat quickly.

Start making nutrient-dense smoothies by checking out the next chapters where you will get delicious smoothie recipes that will help improve your metabolism and keep your energy high.

You will learn what role detoxification plays in weight loss and how you can make detox smoothies at home. I encourage you to discover in the final chapters of this book a simple and effective kick-start plan for your weight loss journey. A daily routine plan that offers an optimal combination of exercise routine, smoothie diet, and your main check-ins to monitor the results.

Chapter 3
Smoothie Recipes for Weight Loss

The most exciting part of this book is here! In this chapter, you will find 30 amazing smoothie recipes that are full of nutrients and are delicious, yet simple.

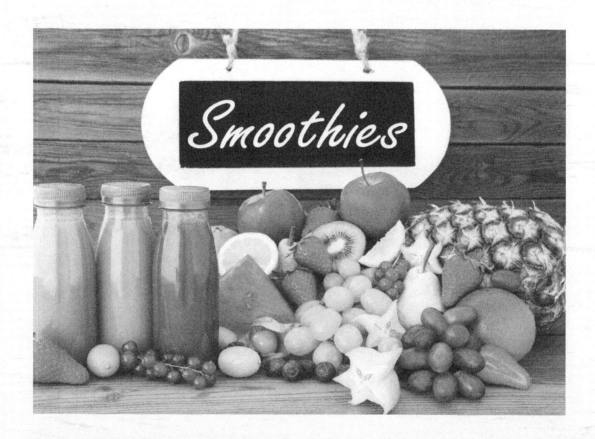

Get our new release for FREE!

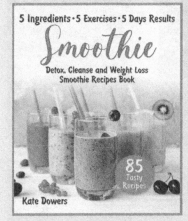
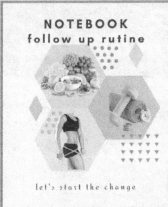

Sing up to our newsletter to get the future release absolutely Free!

https://mailchi.mp/b7abe36ee0fc/kate-dowers

Strawberry-Banana

Strawberries and bananas smoothie—this is a classic combination. It is creamy, sweet, and made from fresh ingredients. Both strawberries and bananas are full of antioxidants, fiber, and nutrients to give your body that extra kick. You can have this smoothie as your morning quick breakfast and it will help fuel your body with much-needed energy.

Ingredients :

- *2 cups frozen strawberries, cut in half*
- *1 frozen banana*
- *½ cup Greek yogurt*
- *½ cup milk (plant-based or regular)*

Nutritional :

- Total Fat: 7.1 g
- Carbohydrates: 31 g
- Dietary fiber: 30.8 g
- Total sugars: 20.5 g
- Protein : 5.9 g
- Calcium : 99 mg
- Potassium : 467 mg
- Cholesterol : 21 mg

2 cups   **5 mins**   **198.1 kcal**

*Blend all the ingredients into your blender for 30 seconds or until smooth. Divide it into two cups and enjoy!

Peanut Butter Banana

Peanut butter banana smoothie is a delicious blend of ingredients. Packed with nutrients, this smoothie just requires 5 ingredients to prepare. You can add some more ingredients like protein powder, chocolate chips, spinach, or kale if you like and make it more nutritious.

Ingredients :

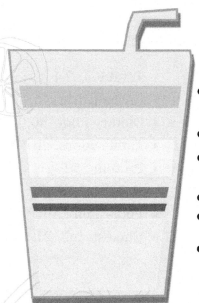

- *2 Tbsp peanut butter (all-natural)*
- *½ cup Greek yogurt*
- *1 cup almond milk (sugar-free)*
- *½ ground flax seeds*
- *1 tsp. vanilla extract*

- *2 cups frozen bananas*

Nutritional :

- Total Fat: 10 g
- Carbohydrates: 40 g
- Dietary fiber: 6 g
- Total sugars: 21 g
- Protein : 12 g
- Calcium : 179 mg
- Potassium : 359 mg
- Cholesterol : 21.2 mg

2 cups   *10 mins*   *295 kcal*

*Blend all the ingredients into your blender until smooth.

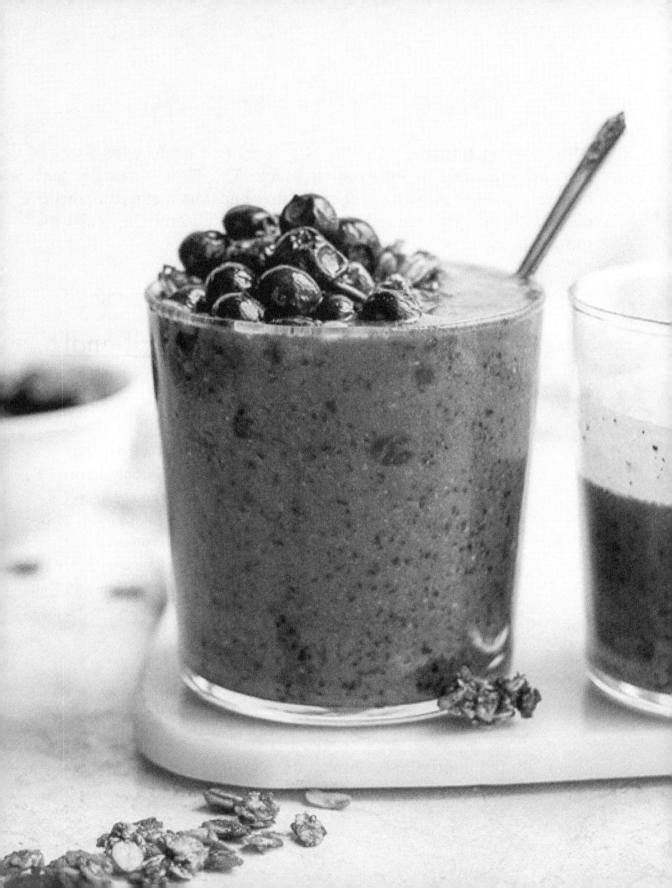

Blueberry Banana

<u>Blueberry & Banana</u> smoothie is creamy and perfect for a quick morning breakfast or an evening snack. The fiber, vitamins, and minerals present in both blueberries and bananas make it a power-packed combo. This smoothie will keep you full and energized for the whole day.

Ingredients :

Nutritional :

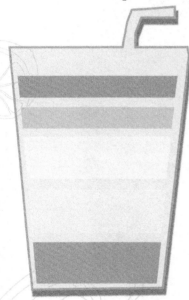

- **1 teaspoon vanilla extract**
- **1 tablespoon flax meal**
- **1 cup unsweetened almond milk**
- **1 cup frozen sliced bananas**
- **1 cup frozen blueberries**

- Total Fat: 3 g
- Carbohydrates: 29 g
- Dietary fiber: 5 g
- Total sugars: 17 g
- Protein : 3 g
- Calcium : 156 mg
- Potassium : 182 mg
- Cholesterol : 0 mg

2 cups   **5 mins**   **147 kcal**

*Blend all the ingredients into your blender until smooth. If the mixture is thick, add some almond milk.

Apple Beetroot Carrot

Apple Beetroot Carrot smoothie is full of antioxidants, vitamins, and minerals but low in calories. It has various digestive, anti-inflammatory, and immune-boosting properties, which makes it the perfect energy booster.

Ingredients :

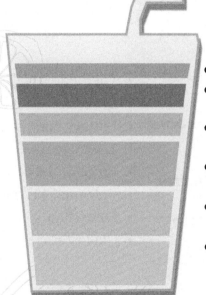

- *1 2-inch fresh ginger*
- *1 red beet cut into chunks*
- *1 apple cut into chunks*
- *3 carrots cut into chunks*
- *juice of 1 orange*

- *1 cup cold water*

Nutritional :

- Total Fat: 1 g
- Carbohydrates: 33 g
- Dietary fiber: 7 g
- Total sugars: 23 g
- Protein : 2 g
- Calcium : 68 mg
- Potassium : 642 mg
- Cholesterol : 0 mg

2 cups   10mins   134 kcal

*Blend all the ingredients into your blender until smooth. Separate into two cups and enjoy!

Coconut Cashew Protein

<u>Coconut Cashew protein</u> smoothie is a staple for weight loss because it comprises just the right amount of fat, protein, and carbs which keep your blood sugar levels in check, and that results in the secretion of a fat-burning hormone called glucagon from the pancreas.

Ingredients :

- **½ banana**
- **¼ cup full-fat coconut milk**
- **1 Tbsp cashew butter**
- **2 scoops of protein powder**
- **2-3 ice cubes**

Nutritional :

- Total Fat: 21 g
- Carbohydrates: 26 g
- Dietary fiber: 4 g
- Total sugars: 9 g
- Protein : 14 g
- Calcium : 112 mg
- Potassium : 556 mg
- Cholesterol : 0 mg

 2 cups   **5 mins**   **315 kcal**

*Blend all the ingredients into your blender until smooth, split, and enjoy!

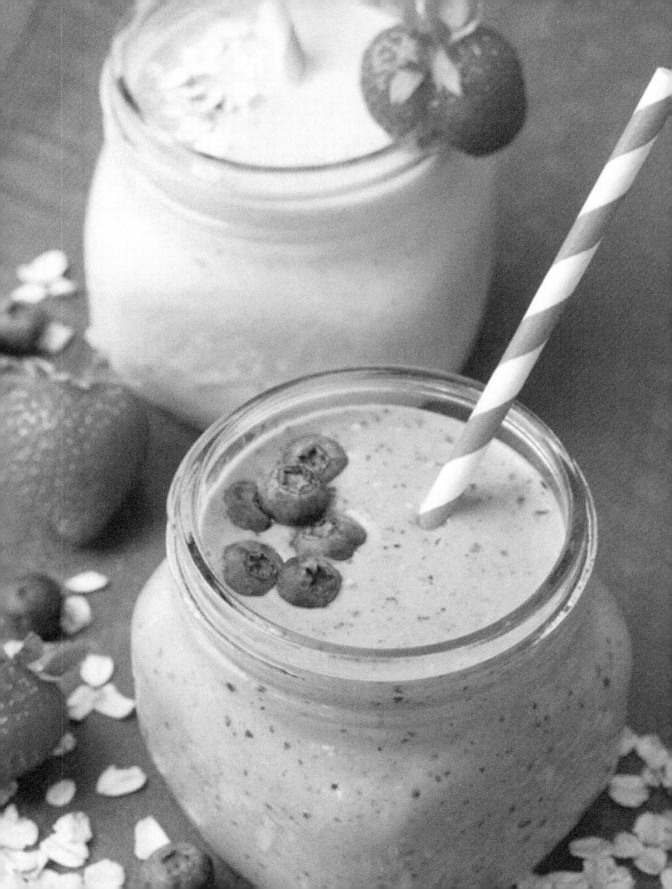

Berry Oat

Berry Oat smoothie has highly nutritious blueberries and oats to ensure you stay full till lunchtime. If you are not fond of having oats as a meal, blend them up in a smoothie! Just make sure to use fresh ingredients.

Ingredients :

Nutritional :

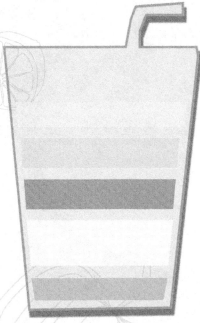

- *⅓ cup vanilla or Greek yogurt*
- *½ cup old fashioned rolled oats*
- *½ cup frozen berries (any berries)*

- *1 cup milk*

- *¼ cup ice*

- Total Fat: 49 g
- Carbohydrates: 32 g
- Dietary fiber: 33 g
- Total sugars: 35,9 g
- Protein : 10,6 g
- Calcium : 224 mg
- Potassium : 361 mg
- Cholesterol : 0 mg

2 cups   *5 mins*   **280 kcal**

*Blend all the ingredients into your blender until smooth, split, and enjoy!

Carrot Cake

Carrot Cake smoothie is rich in polyunsaturated fatty acids. The walnuts present in the smoothie increase diet-induced calorie burn and metabolic rate. They have more omega-3 fatty acids than other nuts. Bonus: One cup of the smoothie can suffice one day's need for Vitamin.

Ingredients :

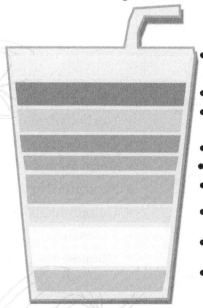

- *9 oz vanilla or Greek yogurt*
- *1/4 cup walnuts*
- *1/4 cup shredded coconut*
- *1/4 tsp ground ginger*
- *1/2 tsp ground cinnamon*
- *4 medium carrots*
- *1 Tbs honey*
- *1 cup almond milk*
- *½ cup ice (optional)*

Nutritional :

- Total Fat: 49 g
- Carbohydrates: 32 g
- Dietary fiber: 33 g
- Total sugars: 35,9 g
- Protein : 10,6 g
- Calcium : 224 mg
- Potassium : 361 mg
- Cholesterol : 0 mg

2 cups   **5 mins**   **280 kcal**

*Blend all the ingredients until ingredients into your blender until smooth. Separate into two cups.

Strawberry Acai

Strawberry Acai smoothie is simple, tasty, and very quick to make. Just throw in a packet of frozen acai, strawberries, banana, and plant milk to a blender, and you will get a refreshing smoothie full of vitamins.

Ingredients :

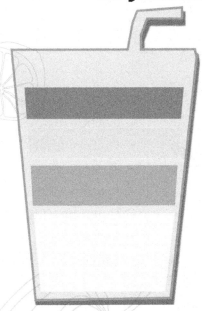

- *3.5 oz packet frozen acai*
- *1 banana*
- *1 cup strawberries*
- *3/4 cup almond milk or cashew milk*

Nutritional :

- Total Fat: 2 g
- Carbohydrates: 25 g
- Dietary fiber: 3 g
- Total sugars: 15 g
- Protein : 1 g
- Calcium : 137 mg
- Potassium : 321 mg
- Cholesterol : 0 mg

 2 cups *3 mins*   *118 kcal*

*Blend all the ingredients into your blender until smooth. Separate into two cups and enjoy!

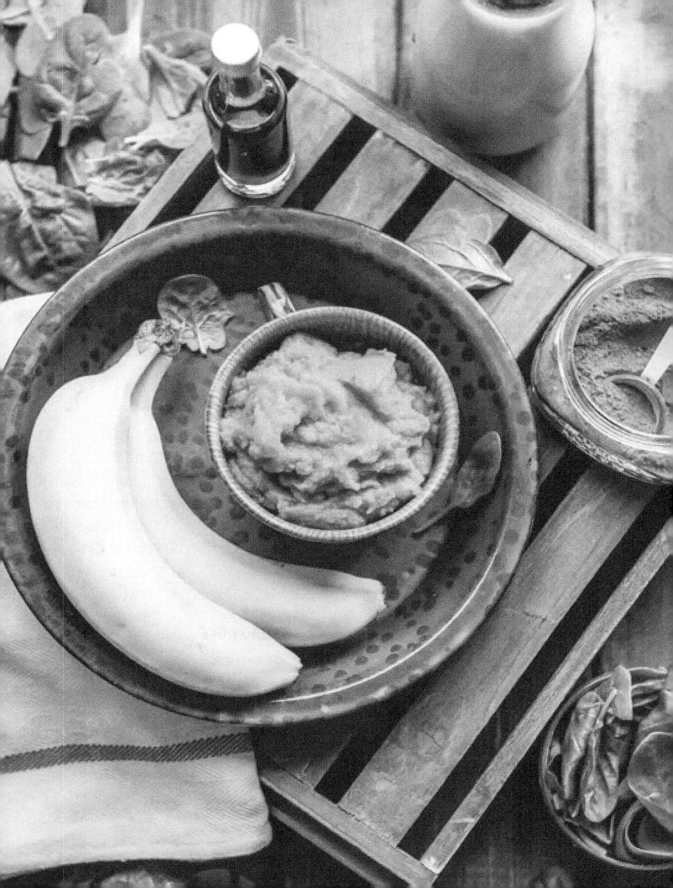

Pumpkin Spice

Pumpkin smoothie is a healthy version of a latte made with pumpkin puree, coffee, frozen banana, and pumpkin pie spice! Pumpkin is rich in many antioxidants, vitamins, and minerals that support your immune system. The coffee added gives in some flavor and also provides you the energy needed for the day.

Ingredients :

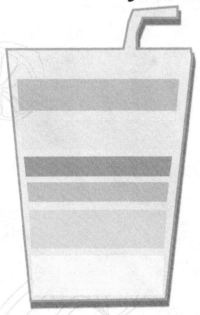

- *1/2 cup unsweetened pumpkin puree*
- *2 frozen banana*
- *1 teaspoon maple syrup*
- *1/2 teaspoon pumpkin pie spice*
- *3/4 cup coffee, cold*
- *3/4 cup milk, any kind*

Nutritional :

- Total Fat: 2 g
- Carbohydrates: 38 g
- Dietary fiber: 5 g
- Total sugars: 20 g
- Protein : 3 g
- Calcium : 116 mg
- Potassium : 256 mg
- Cholesterol : 0 mg

2 cups   *5 mins*   **171 kcal**

*Blend all the ingredients into your blender for 1 minute or until smooth, divide into two cups and enjoy!

Blackberry Cinnamon

Blackberry Cinnamon, this healthy smoothie contains a bunch of apples, blackberries, bananas, dates, and vanilla. The addition of cinnamon and yogurt makes your smoothie more delicious and thick. Moreover, dates—the ultimate sweetener—shapes this smoothie into a healthy and yummy treat!

Ingredients :

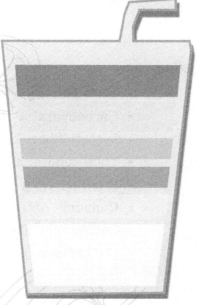

- **1 cup frozen blackberries**
- **1 frozen banana**

- **1 small apple diced**
- **2 dried dates pitted**
- **½ cup vanilla yogurt**

- **1 cup unsweetened vanilla almond milk or milk**

! Optional: 1 Tbs ground flaxseed meal, 2 Tsp ground cinnamon, ½ Tsp pure vanilla extract.

Nutritional :

- Total Fat: 1,5 g
- Carbohydrates: 42 g
- Dietary fiber: 93 g
- Total sugars: 26,8 g
- Protein : 55 g
- Calcium : 160 mg
- Potassium : 602 mg
- Cholesterol : 4 mg

2 cups   5 mins   218 kcal

*Blend all the ingredients into your blender until smooth.

Green Pomegranate

Pomegranate Green Smoothie bowl works great as your breakfast replacement. Made with tons of delicious and healthy ingredients: pomegranate juice, frozen fruits, kale, and protein powder, this smoothie can be your go-to breakfast. Don't like kale? You won't even notice it's there.

Ingredients :

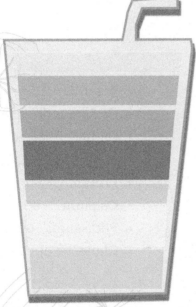

- *1 frozen banana, medium*
- *1/2 cup frozen strawberries*
- *1 cup fresh kale*
- *1/2 cup pomegranate juice*
- *1 scoop vanilla protein powder*
- *1/2 cup Greek yogurt*
- *1/2 cup water*

Nutritional :

- Total Fat: 2 g
- Carbohydrates: 39 g
- Dietary fiber: 2,8 g
- Total sugars: 28 g
- Protein : 1,6 g
- Calcium : 555 mg
- Potassium : 471 mg
- Cholesterol : 0 mg

! Ttoppings: pistachio nuts, hemp seeds, pomegranate arils, and dark chocolate (or whatever you have at home)

2 cups   **5 mins**   **210 kcal**

*Blend all the ingredients into your blender for 1 minute or until smooth, divide into two cups and enjoy!

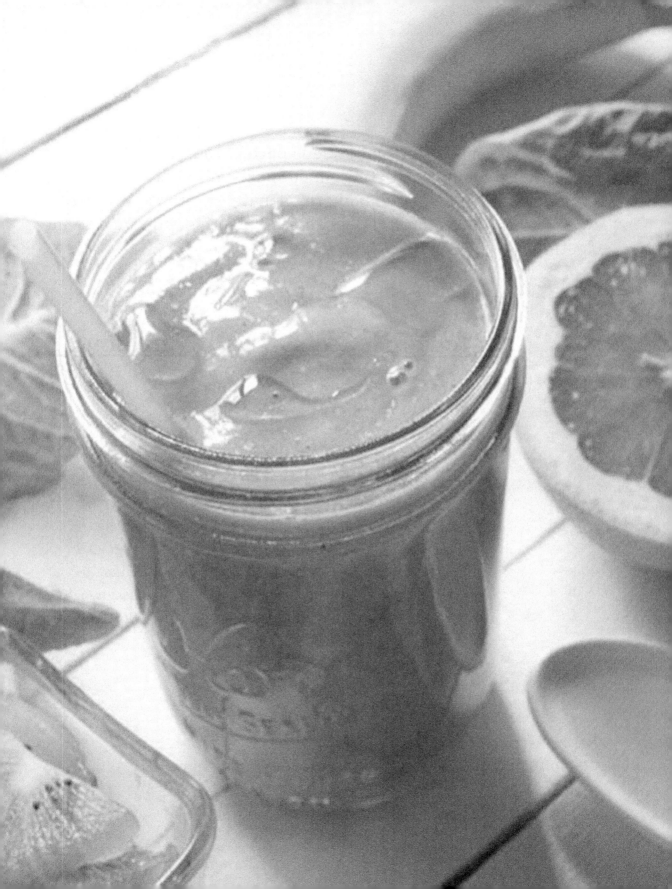

Kiwi Basil

This cool and refreshing smoothie is perfect to have by the beach. Made of kiwi and basil, this smoothie is filled with nutrients, vitamin C, which helps the body rejuvenate. For those who have a sweet tooth, the natural sugars in the smoothie won't cause any bloating, so you can have it guilt-free.

Ingredients :

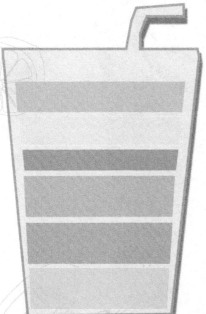

- *3 frozen kiwis*
- *1 banana*
- *1 tbsp agave syrup*
- *1 pink grapefruit juice*
- *a handful of fresh basil*
- *a handful of ice cubes*

Nutritional :

- Total Fat: 1,8 g
- Carbohydrates: 91 g
- Dietary fiber: 12 g
- Total sugars: 46,8 g
- Protein : 5,2 g
- Calcium : 51 mg
- Potassium : 433 mg
- Cholesterol : 0 mg

 2 cups   **5 mins**   **365 kcal**

*Blend! Blend! Blend! Separate into two cups and enjoy!

Almond Orange

It is a five-ingredient, simple yet delicious smoothie that uses seasonal fruits to make a blend packed with nutrients and flavor. The amount of vitamin C and calcium in this smoothie will help fight off the bad guys in your immune system.

Ingredients :

- **4 oranges**
- **1/2 tsp vanilla extract**
- **1 banana**
- **2 tbsp almond butter**
- **1 cup water**

Nutritional :

- Total Fat: 9 g
- Carbohydrates: 50 g
- Dietary fiber: 9 g
- Total sugars: 32 g
- Protein : 1,6 g
- Calcium : 168 mg
- Potassium : 665 mg
- Cholesterol : 0 mg

 2 cups   **10 mins**   **286 kcal**

*Blend! Blend! Blend! Separate into two cups and enjoy!

Vanilla Date Smoothie

Your body often craves a mix of carbohydrates and protein to recover, and this smoothie provides just those. Though the sugar content seems high, it is coming naturally from the fruit. So, unless you have diabetes, you can have this smoothie anytime.

Ingredients :

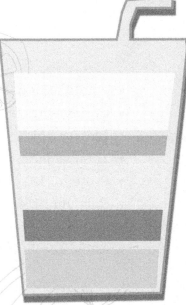

- *1 cup unsweetened almond milk*
- *1 tsp vanilla extract*

- *1 large frozen banana*

- *4 average dates, pitted*
- *5 ice cubes*

Nutritional :

- Total Fat: 5 g
- Carbohydrates: 74 g
- Dietary fiber: 8 g
- Total sugars: 48 g
- Protein : 28 g
- Calcium : 378 mg
- Potassium : 670 mg
- Cholesterol : 0 mg

 1 cups   *10 mins*   *443 kcal*

*Blend all the ingredients into your blender until smooth.

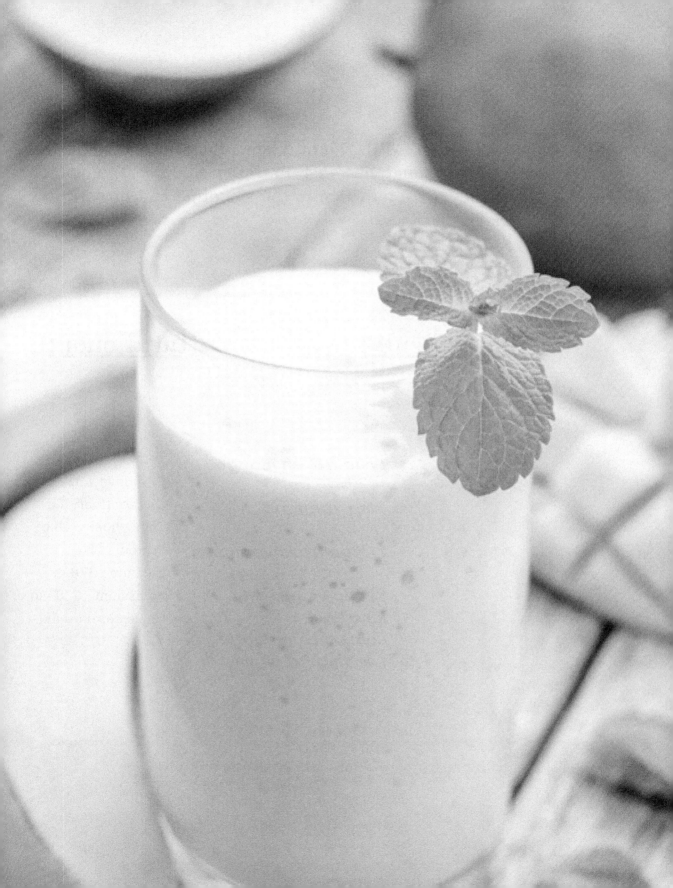

Golden Milk Mango

This nutrient-**Golden Milk Mango** smoothie takes just a few minutes to prepare and has just four ingredients. The add-on turmeric provides extra nutrition to the smoothie and turns it into a golden milkshake.

Ingredients :

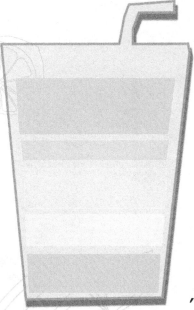

- *1 cup frozen mango*

- *1 tsp turmeric*

- *1 large frozen banana*

- *¾ cup yogurt any kind*
- *some milk or water ,to make the mixture smooth*

Nutritional :

- Total Fat: 5 g
- Carbohydrates: 74 g
- Dietary fiber: 8 g
- Total sugars: 48 g
- Protein : 28 g
- Calcium : 378 mg
- Potassium : 670 mg
- Cholesterol : 0 mg

2 cups   *5 mins*   *443 kcal*

*Blend! Blend! Blend! Separate into two cups and enjoy!

Green Smoothie Recipes

If you want to include more vegetables in your diet, then this section provides all the best green smoothie recipes. You can choose your favorites and have them rotationally to fulfill your daily green intake.

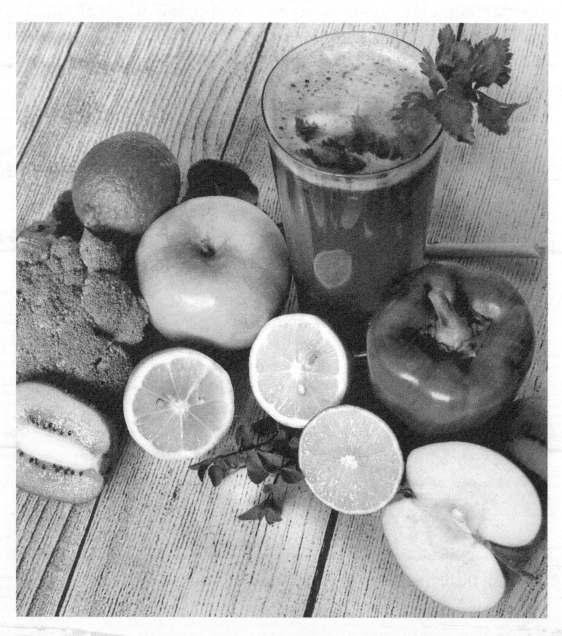

Classic Green

The list cannot be complete without a **Classic Green** Smoothie addition when it comes to green smoothies. This wholesome smoothie contains bananas, apples, and spinach, all of which are rich in fiber, vitamin C, antioxidants, and other nutrients. Adding them together is the perfect way to get some greens in your body.

Ingredients :

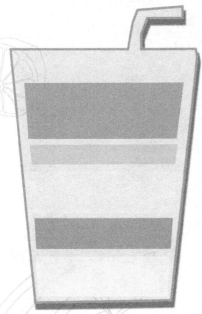

- *2 cups spinach*
- *1/4 avocado*
- *1 large frozen banana*
- *1 apple*
- *1-1/2 cup vegans milk or regular milk*

Nutritional :

- Total Fat: 5 g
- Carbohydrates: 29 g
- Dietary fiber: 6 g
- Total sugars: 17 g
- Protein : 3 g
- Calcium : 260 mg
- Potassium : 657 mg
- Cholesterol : 0 mg

 2 cups   *5 mins*   *163 kcal*

*Blend all the ingredients into your blender until smooth.

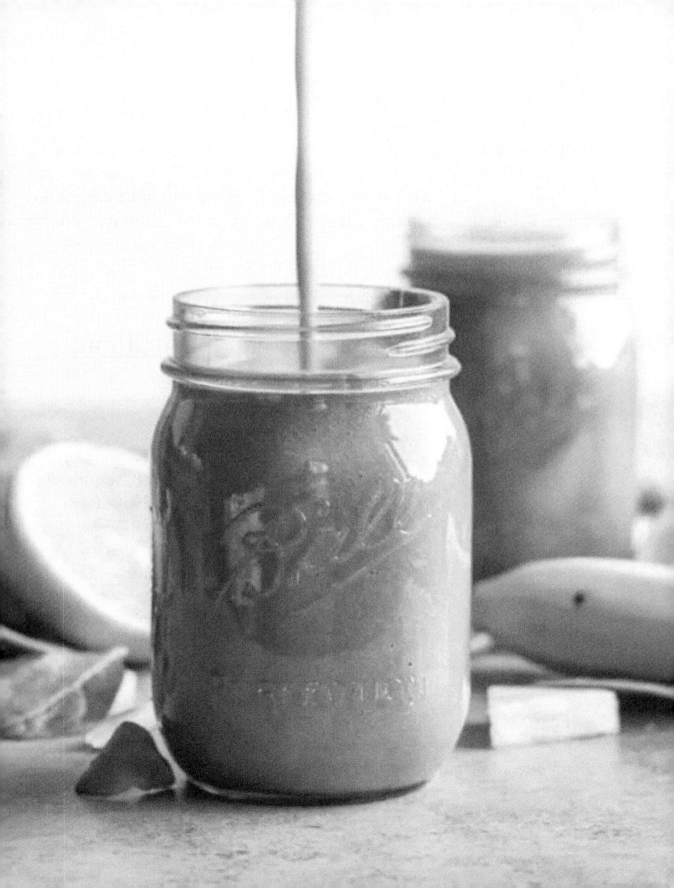

Tropical Green

Tropical Green Smoothie is full of antioxidants and Vitamin C. The matcha green tea in the smoothie improves your metabolism and speeds up the weight loss process. If you are looking for an energy drink that gives you tropical vibes in the summer, go for this one.

Ingredients :

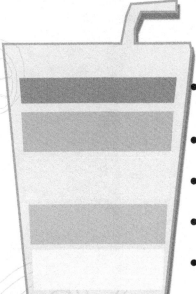

- *2 tbsp matcha green tea powder*
- *½ cup frozen mango*
- *½ frozen banana*
- *½ cup orange juice*
- *½ cup coconut milk*

Nutritional :

- Total Fat: 33 g
- Carbohydrates: 32 g
- Dietary fiber: 16 g
- Total sugars: 14 g
- Protein : 9 g
- Calcium : 116 mg
- Potassium : 678 mg
- Cholesterol : 0 mg

2 cups *10 mins* *321kcal*

*Blend! Blend! Blend! Separate into two cups and enjoy!

Kale Recharge Smoothie

Kale Recharge Smoothie is full of vitamin A and antioxidants and is also low in calories. It is perfect for people trying to get some extra greens but is not a fan of eating raw kale because you can't taste it among the other amazing flavors.

Ingredients :

- *1 Tbsp fresh parsley*
- *¾ cups curly kale*
- *¾ cup spinach,*
- *1 frozen ripe banana*
- *1 tsp lime juice*
- *1 tsp ginger, grated*
- *½ cup carrots*
- *8 oz' water*
- *4 ice cubes*

Nutritional :

- Total Fat: 0 g
- Carbohydrates: 14 g
- Dietary fiber: 3 g
- Total sugars: 5 g
- Protein : 2 g
- Calcium : 54 mg
- Potassium : 769 mg
- Cholesterol : 0 mg

1 cups   **5 mins**   **58 kcal**

*Blend all the ingredients into your blender until smooth.

Green Veggie

The **Green Veggie** smoothie is an ideal smoothie for your daily green intake. It has higher nutritional value and has a refreshing taste. Take a look at the ingredients needed.

Ingredients :

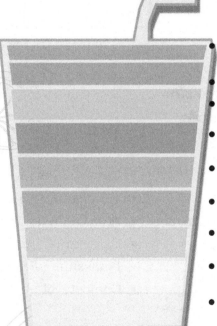

- **A few basil and curry leaves**
- **A handful coriander**
- **1 cup spinach**
- **1 green cucumber**
- **½ cup mint leaves**
- **2 tbsp bottle gourd**
- **2-3 stalks celery**
- **½ cup pineapple**
- **1 lemon for lemon juice**

Nutritional :

- Total Fat: 0,9 g
- Sodium : 245 mg
- Carbohydrates: 32 g
- Dietary fiber: 7,2 g
- Total sugars: 16,2g
- Protein : 5,4 g
- Calcium : 365 mg
- Potassium : 1143 mg
- Cholesterol : 0 mg

2 cups   **5 mins**   **134 kcal**

*Blend all the ingredients into your blender until smooth.

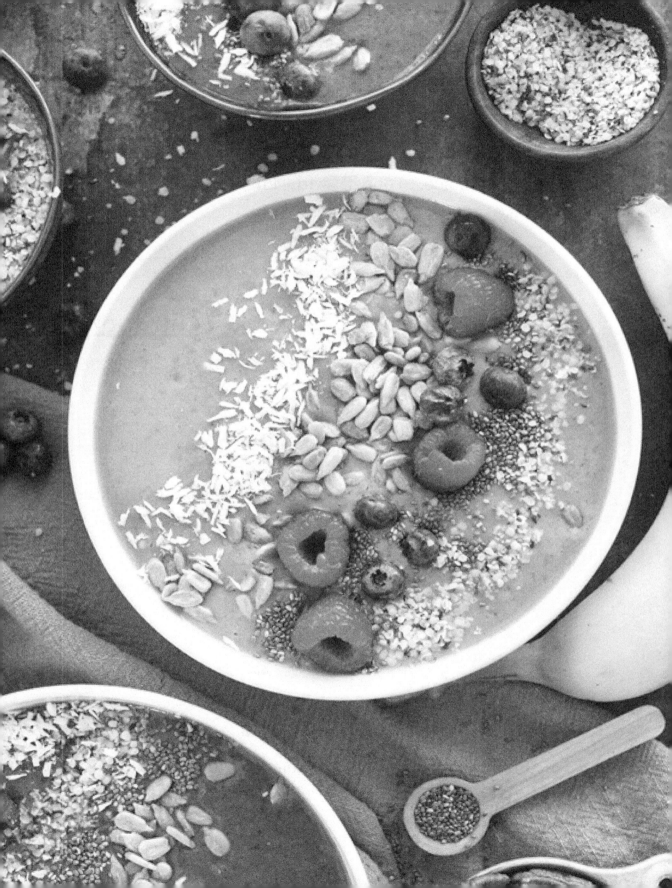

Clean Green Smoothie

If you want a replacement in your fairy greens smoothie, this one is a perfect choice. Topped with kiwis and blueberries, this smoothie is a wonderful win.

Ingredients :

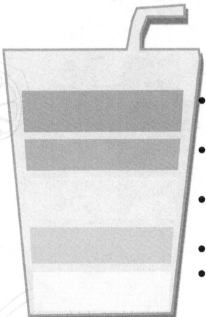

- **2 cups of spinach (or other leafy green)**
- **1/2 cup blueberries**

- **2 bananas, sliced and frozen**
- **1/2 avocado**
- **1 cup coconut water (or plain water)**

Nutritional :

- Total Fat: 20 g
- Carbohydrates: 59 g
- Dietary fiber: 14 g
- Total sugars: 30 g
- Protein : 8 g
- Calcium : 109 mg
- Potassium : 1568 mg
- Cholesterol : 0 mg

! Toppings: 2 kiwi fruit, peeled and sliced, 2 tbsp sunflower seeds, 1/4 cup coconut flakes

2 cups   **5 mins**   **420 kcal**

---

*Blend all the ingredients into your blender until smooth. Pour into two bowls and top it with some mixed fruit and seeds, including.

Avocado-Lime Green Tea

The Avocado present in the smoothie contains healthy fats, which help to soak other nutrients. This one is a bit high on the ingredients, but that is great to include if you are on a cleansing diet. It also helps in keeping the immune system strong that helps fight off various infections and diseases.

Ingredients :

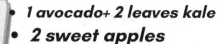

- *1 avocado+ 2 leaves kale*
- *2 sweet apples*
- *1 small knob ginger*
- *½ cup chopped broccoli*
- *½ small zucchini*
- *¼ cup parsley*
- *½ juiced lime*
- *1 cup cold green tea*
- *⅔ cup almond milk*

Nutritional :

- Total Fat: 20,8 g
- Carbohydrates: 44 g
- Dietary fiber: 13,3 g
- Total sugars: 21,3 g
- Protein : 5 g
- Calcium : 29 mg
- Potassium : 598 mg
- Cholesterol : 0 mg

2 cups   **10 mins**   **365 kcal**

*Blend all the ingredients into your blender until smooth. Separate into two servings and enjoy!

Mango and Hemp Seeds

This green smoothie is the seasonal version of the original recipe, including fall fruits like apples, cinnamon, and hemp flax seeds. It can be the perfect replacement for your daily nutritional meal. The fall flavors can be swapped with seasonal fruits and cinnamon with alternative flavors.

Ingredients :

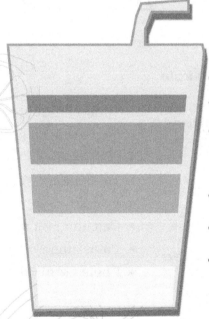

- *⅛ teaspoon sea salt*
- *2 Tbsp hemp seeds*
- *3 handfuls baby kale {or spinach}*
- *1/2 cup mango, diced*
- *1 banana*
- *1/2 cup unsweet almond milk*

Nutritional :

- Total Fat: 9,3 g
- Carbohydrates: 62 g
- Dietary fiber: 8,4 g
- Total sugars: 25,7 g
- Protein : 13,5 g
- Calcium : 445 mg
- Potassium : 1783 mg
- Cholesterol : 0 mg

1 cups   *2 mins*   **358 kcal**

*Blend all the ingredients into your blender until smooth. Pour into a bowl and top it with mixed fruits.

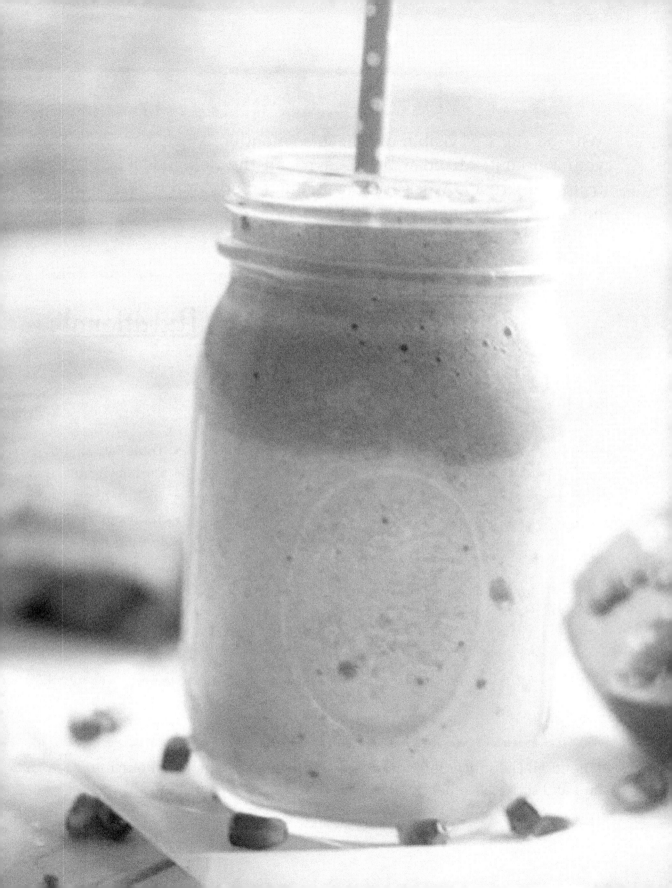

Strawberry Pomegranate

With no signs of visible green, this smoothie is great to have after your workout. Mixed with spinach and the deliciousness of other fruits, this recipe will satisfy your taste buds and give you all the nutritional value needed for the body.

Ingredients :

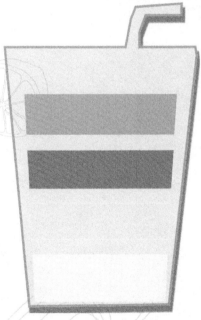

- **1 cup fresh spinach**

- **1/4 cup pomegranate seeds**
- **1/2 frozen banana**

- **1/4 cup coconut water**

Nutritional :

- Total Fat: 25,4 g
- Carbohydrates: 68 g
- Dietary fiber: 10,5 g
- Total sugars: 38,3 g
- Protein : 6 g
- Calcium : 103 mg
- Potassium : 1200 mg
- Cholesterol : 0 mg

! **For pink layer**: 1 frozen banana, 1/2 cup coconut water, 1 cup frozen strawberries (or fresh!).

1 cups   **5 mins**   **483 kcal**

*Blend all the ingredients into your blender until smooth. Pour into a jar or cup and top it with berries.

Green Warrior Protein

It is a supercharged smoothie in a glass. You can use hemp hearts as the major protein source for your smoothie. It also contains omega 3-6-9 fatty acids and fiber. This smoothie is extra creamy without using extra bananas.

Ingredients :

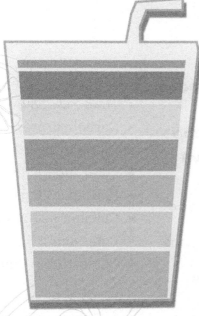

- **3 tablespoons hemp**
- **1 cup kale or baby spinach**
- **1 medium celery stalk**
- **1 large sweet apple**
- **1 cup chopped cucumber**
- **1/3 cup frozen mango**
- **1/2 cup fresh red grapefruit juice**

Nutritional :

- Total Fat: 7 g
- Carbohydrates: 29 g
- Dietary fiber: 6 g
- Total sugars: 15 g
- Protein : 7 g
- Calcium : 6 mg
- Potassium : 130 mg
- Cholesterol : 0 mg

! Optional: 1 tsp virgin coconut oil, 2 tablespoons fresh mint leaves, 4 ice cubes, or as needed

3 cups   10 mins   200 kcal

*Blend all the ingredients into your blender until smooth.

Mango Coconut Green

Due to the coconut milk base, this smoothie is vegan and extra smooth, and creamy. This green glass of smoothie has a coconutty and creamy flavor while the. Mango gives it a fruity vibe that gives you a beachy vibe.

Ingredients :

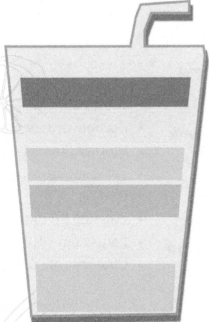

- **1 cup fresh washed spinach leaves**
- **1/2 medium banana**
- **1 cup fresh /frozen mango cubes**
- **1/2 cup orange juice**
- **3/4 cup coconut milk**
- **1/2 cup ice cubes**

Nutritional :

- Total Fat: 18 g
- Carbohydrates: 28 g
- Dietary fiber: 2,7 g
- Total sugars: 20,1 g
- Protein : 3,6 g
- Calcium : 27 mg
- Potassium : 555 mg
- Cholesterol : 0 mg

1 cups   **5 mins**   **273 kcal**

*Blend all the ingredients into your blender until smooth.

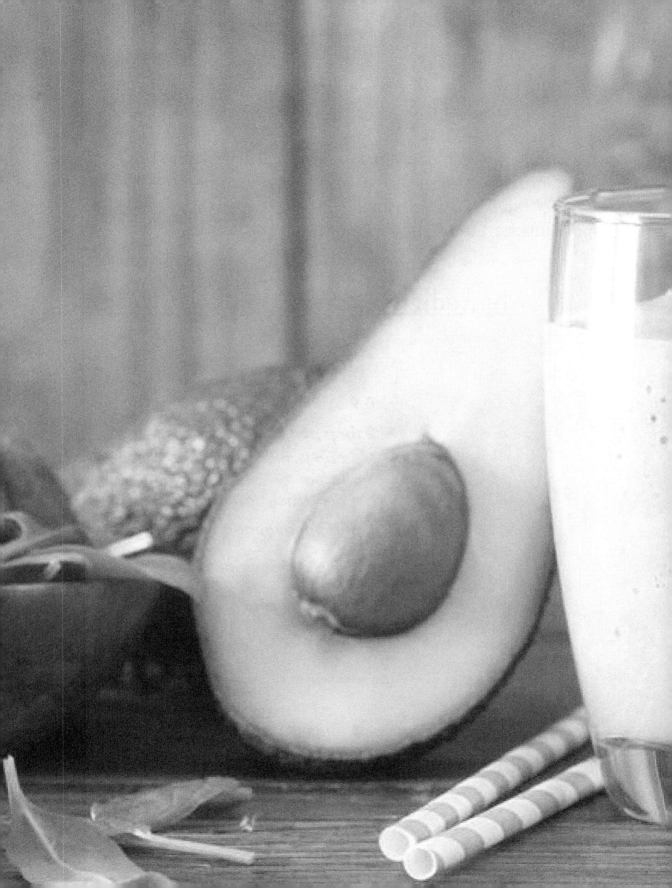

Low Carb Shamrock Protein

If you are not a smoothie fan, you will love this recipe. It can be your breakfast alternative and some people also prefer it for Easter and St. Patrick's Day. It is high in fiber and monounsaturated fat and potassium.

Ingredients :

- **0,9 oz Powder NuZest**
- **2 tbsp pistachio nuts**
- **1/4 cup vanilla or collagen**
- **1/4 cup fresh spinach**
- **1 medium avocado**
- **1/4 cup coconut milk**
- **1/2 cup of water**

Nutritional :

- Total Fat: 37,1 g
- Carbohydrates: 9,1 g
- Dietary fiber: 10,9 g
- Total sugars: 3,1g
- Protein : 27,1 g
- Calcium : 33 mg
- Potassium : 959 mg
- Cholesterol : 0 mg

! **Topping :** 3-6 drops liquid stevia, 1/2 vanilla bean or 1 tsp sugar-free vanilla extract, fresh mint /mint extract

1 cups   **5 mins**   **493 kcal**

*Blend! Blend! Blend! Put ice cubes and enjoy!

Snickerdoodle Green

This **Snickerdoodle Green** smoothie is extra smooth and has a delicious taste. When mixed with avocado, cinnamon, and vanilla, it tastes like a snickerdoodle cookie.

Ingredients :

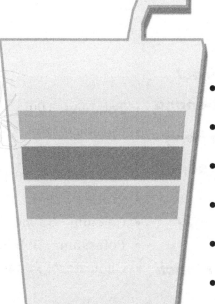

- *1/2 tsp vanilla*
- *1/4 tsp cinnamon*
- *1 handful spinach*
- *1/2 small avocado*
- *1 frozen banana*
- *1/4 cup almond milk*

Nutritional :

- Total Fat: 4,4 g
- Carbohydrates: 38 g
- Dietary fiber: 11 g
- Total sugars: 15,3 g
- Protein : 4,3 g
- Calcium : 129 mg
- Potassium : 1130 mg
- Cholesterol : 0 mg

1 cups   **5 mins**   **334 kcal**

*Blend all the ingredients into your blender until smooth. Serve with ice.

Tropical Green

This healthy green smoothie has a delicious taste that gives you the vibe of virgin pina colada and the nutritions of healthy greens. All ingredients may be frozen as well as fresh.

Ingredients :

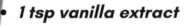

- 1 tsp vanilla extract
- 1 medium ripe banana
- 1 cup a favorite berry
- 1 cup frozen pineapple chunks
- 1 cup frozen mango chunks
- 2 cups frozen spinach
- 1 cup milk

Nutritional :

- Total Fat: 10 g
- Carbohydrates:152 g
- Dietary fiber: 26 g
- Total sugars: 10,1g
- Protein : 29 g
- Calcium : 33 mg
- Potassium : 959 mg
- Cholesterol : 0 mg

1 cups   5 mins   743 kcal

*Blend all the ingredients into your blender until smooth.

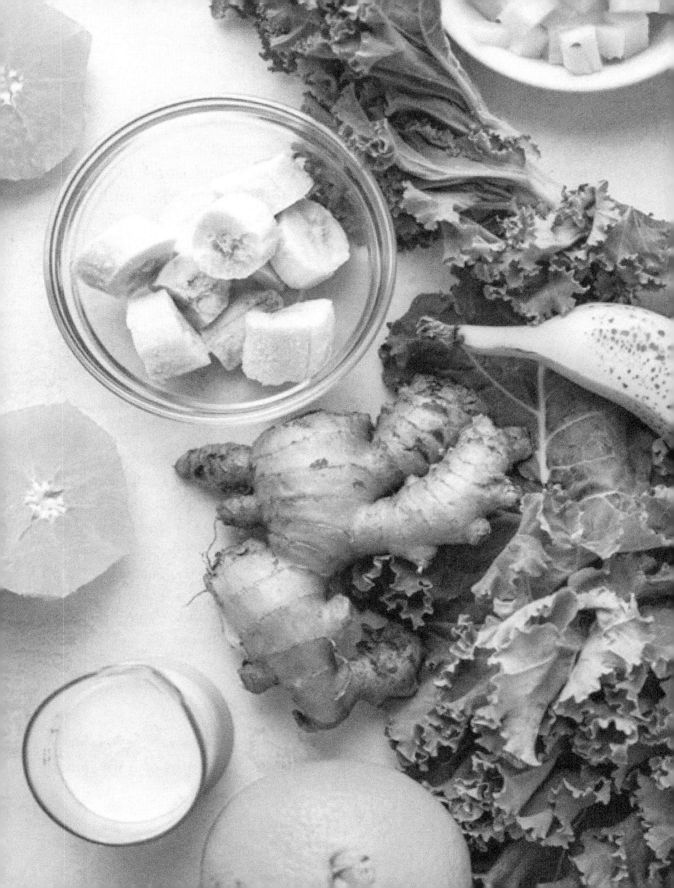

Ginger Green Citrus

Ginger Green Citrus Smoothie is a refreshing smoothie. This smoothie is rich in vitamins with citrus additions like orange, lemon, and apples. Besides being delicious, ginger and spinach give you an extra dose of nutrients and a metabolic boost.

Ingredients :

- *1 Tbp fresh cut ginger*
- *2 hand of spinach*
- *½ frozen banana*
- *1 orange, peeled and cut*
- *1/2 apple, sliced*
- *juice from of 1 lemon*
- *1/2 cup unsweet milk*

Nutritional :

- Total Fat: 1,1 g
- Carbohydrates: 67 g
- Dietary fiber: 10,9 g
- Total sugars: 43,4 g
- Protein : 3,8 g
- Calcium : 86 mg
- Potassium : 947 mg
- Cholesterol : 0 mg

 1 cups   **5 mins**   **268 kcal**

*Blend all the ingredients into your blender for 2 minutes or until smooth.

Blueberry & Peanut Butter

Blueberry & Peanut Butter Green smoothie is a combination of delicious, healthy, and satisfying. This recipe has to redeem powers as well. With a few ingredients, it turns out to be an energy-boosting and tasty smoothie.

Ingredients :

- **1 medium banana**
- **1 cup icy blueberries**
- **1/2 tbsp creamy peanut butter**
- **splash of milk**
- **1-1/2 cups fresh spinach**
- **1/4 cup yogurt**

Nutritional :

- Total Fat: 4,1 g
- Sodium : 81 mg
- Carbohydrates:57 g
- Dietary fiber: 10,6 g
- Total sugars: 33,3g
- Protein : 8,7 g
- Calcium : 214 mg
- Potassium : 929 mg
- Cholesterol : 0 mg

 1 cups   **5 mins**   **277 kcal**

*Blend all the ingredients into your blender until smooth.

Chapter 4
What is Detox? The Importance of Detoxification

Every day, we get exposed to many toxins through the air, water, and food. But, the toxins that harm our body the most are from eating unhealthy food. These foods have high amounts of sugar and other toxic chemicals that slowly deteriorate our bodies and make them full of toxins. Eating processed food regularly can alter the metabolic system of a person and disrupt their hormonal count. Now the question arises: If processed foods are that harmful, why don't people avoid them? It is because the high amount of sugars makes these foods addictive. That's why people can't control consuming them even if they try to.

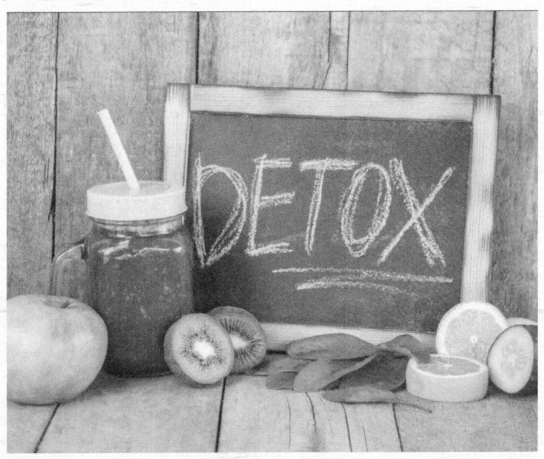

How Toxins Cause Weight Gain

The reason toxins are the major cause of weight gain is that our body fights with these toxins by creating new fat cells. The fat cells trap the toxins to protect your body from poisoning and prevent the toxins from spreading to your main organs. But since the fats cells get developed from the toxins, they fail to perform metabolically. It means that they fail to produce the hormone required for appetite regulation, which results in gaining more weight. Another reason toxin in the body leads to weight gain in the body is that they disturb the working principle of the thyroid gland. Your thyroid gland is responsible for regulating the metabolic rate in your body. If it doesn't function properly, your body's fat-burning process will be slow, and you will not burn as quickly as you could. Toxins also disturb the hormonal balance of your body. The hormones in your body regulate the fat-burning process as well as your hunger levels. Toxins lead to improper hormonal imbalance, which makes it more difficult to lose weight.

Symptoms That Imply Toxins in the Body

Do you often feel tired or stressed? Have you noticed some changes in your body that you have never seen before? If yes, then there might be high chances that your body is suffering from a toxic overload. Toxins are poisonous to your body, and it gives many signs to show you that your toxin levels are high. Here are the most common symptoms that imply you have toxins in your body:

Constipation

The digestive system is responsible for keeping toxins and waste out of your body. Processed foods include harmful chemicals, preservatives, artificial flavors, and colors, which, when consumed, can disturb the digestive system and lead to constipation. As a result, your body faces irregular bowel movements, which results in more fatigue and weakening of the immune system.

Insomnia

Junk and processed foods increase toxin levels that disturb the level of cortisol, a hormone that helps your body deal with stress. The healthy cortisol levels are highest in the morning and lowest in the night. However, if the hormone levels get disturbed, the level can go up even in the evening. It further disturbs your sleep cycle and causes stress.

Skin Issues

Normally, your liver eliminates most of the toxins produced in the body. However, if the amount of toxins gets overloaded, the liver fails to remove them. This results in acne, rashes, and skin inflammation. Other skin conditions that imply the overload of toxins are eczema, swollen eyes, chemical insensitivities, inflammation.

Body Odor and Bad Breath

When the liver fails to get rid of excess toxins from the body, it leads to bad breath and body odor. But, bad breath can also result from a disturbance in the other parts of the body. Bad breath and body odor are the signs that your body is trying to get rid of the toxins in your body.

Muscle Pains

Excess toxins target the pain receptors in your body and lead to muscle pain and knots. The toxins can either have an immediate or aftereffect on your muscles. Increased consumption of fast food builds up the chemicals in your body, weakening your muscles and making you feel lethargic all the time.

Mood Swings

Do you feel stressed and moody all the time? Mood swings indicate hormonal imbalance, and that is a sign of toxin overload. Eating sugary and processed food can result in improper hormonal balance, which affects your mood. The sugar in those foods directly affects your brain and slowly reduces its ability to function. Processed foods also contain toxins like MSG, which affect the brain cells and disturb their functioning.

Feeling Exhausted

If you feel exhausted even after getting the required amount of sleep, chances are you have high levels of toxins in your body. High toxin levels put an extra burden on your adrenal glands, which can cause stress. If the toxic level is high for the long term, it can lead to adrenal fatigue. Adrenal fatigue makes you feel tired and exhausted all the time.

If your body is showing any of these signs, it is high time you detoxify it. Switching to healthy and nutritious food and exercising regularly can ultimately reduce the toxic count in your body. However, if you want to make the process faster, you can start smoothie detoxification. But, first, let us know a little bit about detoxification.

What is Detoxification and Why is it Important?

We all are concerned about our outer cleanliness. We do daily activities like bathing, brushing our teeth, and washing our hair just so they look clean and fresh. While these activities clean our bodies from the outside, detoxification cleanses our bodies from the inside. Detoxification typically refers to following a particular diet to eliminate extra toxins in your body to support weight loss. But, if we dive a little deeper into the concept, we get that our bodies can reduce excess toxins without diets. The body naturally eliminates toxins through the lungs, intestines, kidneys, and lymphatic system. However, when there is a disturbance in these systems, they fail to infiltrate the impurities, leading to an adverse effect on your body. What detoxification does is that it enhances the body's detoxification process. It rejuvenates your body and gives it more strength to five those poisonous toxins.

Our body requires daily vitamins and enzymes to help it get rid of unwanted waste, and to produce those molecules, we need to put healthy foods and supplements in our bodies. When you follow a detoxification diet, your body gets the required amount of nutrients that act as a catalyst for your body to function better. Detoxification is a long-term process that results in cleansing your body and keeping it healthy. Therefore, it is important to adapt to a balanced, healthy diet and eat foods that nourish and replenish your body. If you start right, you will be able to maintain your weight and keep a healthy lifestyle forever. The best way to start detoxifying your body is to add a huge amount of fruits and vegetables to your diet. If you don't like to eat them in chunks, blend them up and make them into a healthy, nutritious smoothie!

Detoxify Your Body with Smoothies

Smoothies are a popular way to give you all the required daily intake of nutrients. Unlike juices, smoothies retain the fiber content of fruits and vegetables that keeps you fuller and more energetic. To make a detox smoothie, you can add tons of nutritional greens like leafy vegetables, celery, and fibrous fruits. You can also go in with some spices to give your smoothie a little kick. Most of us don't consume many fruits and vegetables daily, so smoothies would be the perfect way to blend all that nutrition into your body. The most prominent reason why most people go for a detox smoothie diet is to lose weight. If you do the process right, you can shed as much as 6 pounds a week. A detoxifying smoothie cleanse helps in your digestion, lessen junk food cravings, and the enzymes present in the fruits help shred the extra fat off your body. But to keep your detox smoothie low in calorie and high in nutrition, you need to keep a few things in mind:

●Less sugar: Although fruits add many nutrients, adding many fruits to your smoothie can increase your sugar levels and calorie count. Try adding some greens with your fruits to have a balanced sugar level.

●Healthy fats are your friends: Adding a source of healthy fats such as nut butter or seeds digest your body very slowly and keep your body full.

●Add more protein: Protein deficiency can result in muscle loss instead of weight loss. Therefore, it is crucial to add some protein sources in your smoothies, such as protein powders, dairy, or Greek yogurt, to turn your fat into muscles and prevent it from gaining back.

●And more fiber: Fiber helps in the proper functioning of your digestive system.

To make your smoothie full of fiber, you can add some oats, chia seeds, or flax seeds. Apart from helping you lose weight fast, smoothies also make your skin glow. Adding ingredients high in vitamin C and omega-3 such as flax seeds, avocados, mangoes, lemons, dates are the perfect way to give you glowing skin from within. Besides, adding ingredients rich in melatonin and magnesium such as bananas, honey, almonds, and oats improves your sleep cycle and keeps you stress-free. But, do you know detox smoothies also help in keeping your heart health in check? The next section will provide you with some recipes to detox your heart and keep it healthy.

Tasty Detox Smoothie Recipes

Here are some yummy detox smoothie recipes you can have to shred weight fast.

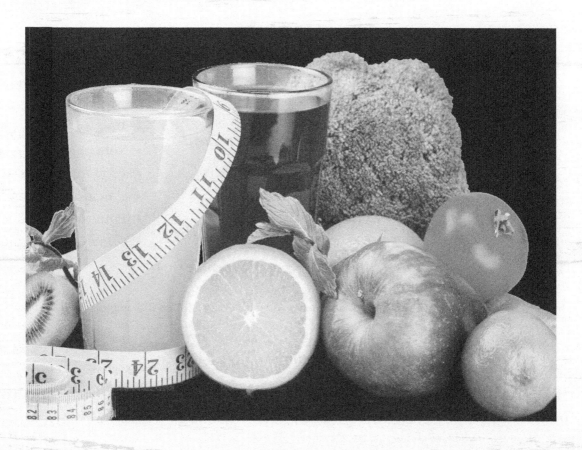

Acai Bowl

This **Acai Bowl** recipe is a perfect blend of antioxidants and has a delicious sweet flavor with various nuts, seeds, berries, keeps, and fruit toppings. It is easy to make and is a great smoothie for your post-workout.

Ingredients :

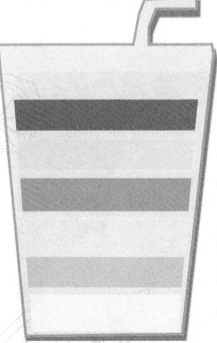

- *2 packets of unsweet frozen acai*
- *1 banana*
- *1 cup frozen mixed berries*
- *1 scoop collagen*
- *2 tbsp almond butter*
- *1 cup cashew milk*

Nutritional :

- Total Fat: 10,7 g
- Sodium : 114 mg
- Carbohydrates: 26 g
- Dietary fiber: 13,9 g
- Total sugars: 13,7g
- Protein : 9,6 g
- Calcium : 335 mg
- Potassium : 543 mg
- Cholesterol : 0 mg

! **Topping:** bee pollen, coconut flakes, chia seeds, mixed berries, optional: hemp seeds, cacao nibs.

2 cups   *5 mins*   **224,6 kcal**

*Blend all the ingredients into your blender until smooth. Pour into two bowls and top it with mixed fruits.

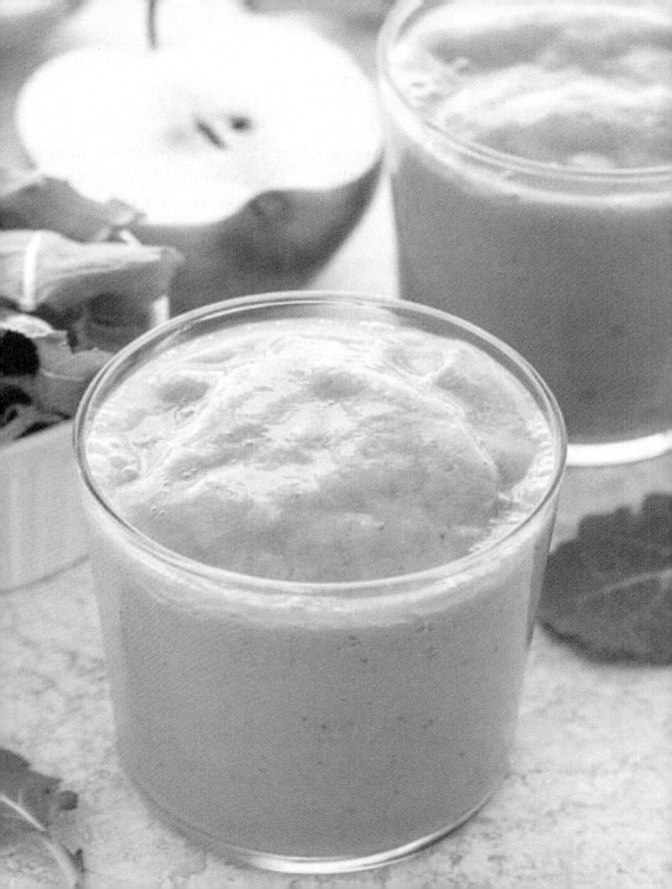

Apple Berry Detox

This **Apple Berry Detox** smoothie recipe is great if you want to improve your metabolism. The vitamins and minerals present in both apples and berries make it a perfect morning refreshment.

Ingredients :

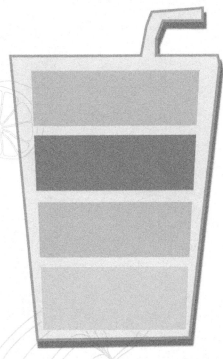

- *1 cup mixed berries*

- *2 cups spinach*

- *1 large apple*

- *1 cup water*

Nutritional :

- Total Fat: 1,1 g
- Sodium: 195 mg
- Carbohydrates: 50 g
- Dietary fiber: 11,7 g
- Total sugars: 7,9 g
- Protein : 3,3 g
- Calcium : 91 mg
- Potassium : 884 mg
- Cholesterol : 0 mg

 1 cups   5 mins   210 kcal

*Blend all the ingredients into your blender until smooth.

Green Detox

Made with some of the most nutritious ingredients on the planet, this smoothie is perfect for your everyday pre-workout session. This smoothie is high in antioxidants, which will give you the ultimate boost for a workout.

Ingredients :

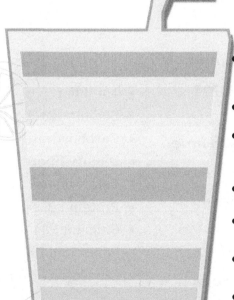

- **a handful of mint leaves**
- **marine salt**
- **1 tbsp sunflower seed powder**
- **1 kiwi**
- **1 celery stick**
- **1/2 avocado**
- **1 cup water**

Nutritional :

- Total Fat: 20,1 g
- Sodium: 195 mg
- Carbohydrates: 21 g
- Dietary fiber: 9,7 g
- Total sugars: 7,1 g
- Protein : 9,6 g
- Calcium : 54 mg
- Potassium : 829 mg
- Cholesterol : 0 mg

1 cups   **5 mins**   **258 kcal**

*Blend! Blend! Blend! And enjoy!

Blood Orange Green

This recipe is simple and quick, requires just 6 ingredients. There is banana, coconut milk, lime juice, blood orange juice, spinach, and kale, making this a smoothie full of benefits. You will get a super creamy, slightly tart smoothie with a lot of vitamins and minerals and without the hint of spinach or kale flavor.

Ingredients :

- **1 frozen banana**
- **2 blood oranges, juiced**
- **2-3 Tbsp fresh lime juice**
- **3/4 cup frozen pineapple**
- **2 handfuls of fresh or frozen greens**
- **3/4 cup coconut milk**

Nutritional :

- Total Fat: 5 g
- Sodium: 48 mg
- Carbohydrates: 32 g
- Dietary fiber: 3 g
- Total sugars: 17,8 g
- Protein : 3,3 g
- Calcium : 84 mg
- Potassium : 870 mg
- Cholesterol : 0 mg

1 cups   **5 mins**   **165 kcal**

*Blend all the ingredients into your blender until smooth. Add ice to get the required consistency.

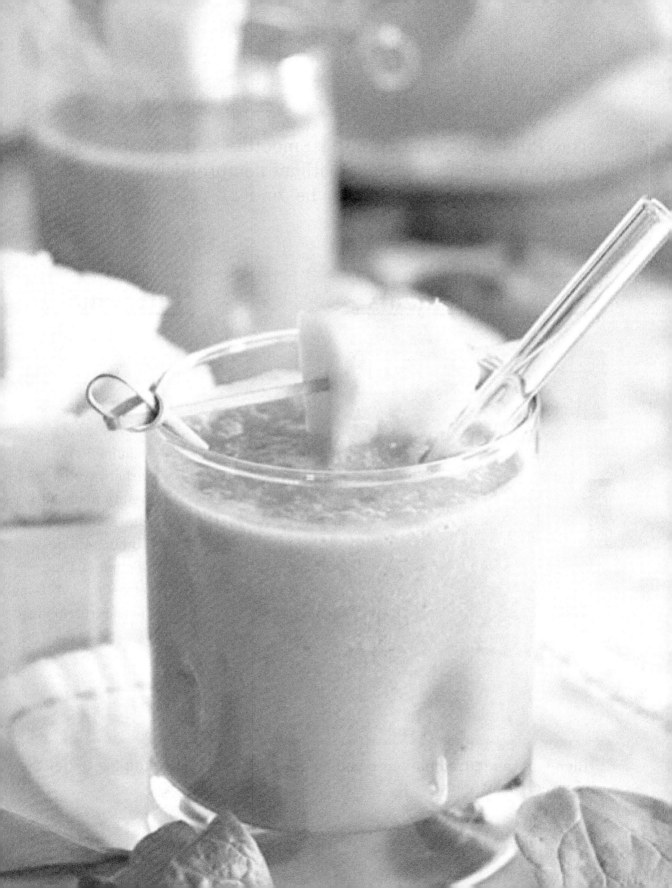

Pineapple Banana Detox

This **Pineapple and Banana** Smoothie is a delicious way to get your daily green intake without compromising taste. Trust me; this recipe is going to be one of your favorite detox smoothie recipes.

Ingredients :

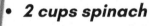

- *2 cups spinach*
- *1 cup pineapple*
- *1 apple*
- *1 banana*
- *1 cup water*

Nutritional :

- Total Fat: 1,2 g
- Sodium: 60 mg
- Carbohydrates: 81 g
- Dietary fiber: 12,1 g
- Total sugars: 54,1 g
- Protein : 4,5 g
- Calcium : 94 mg
- Potassium : 1178 mg
- Cholesterol : 0 mg

1 cups   *5 mins*   **317 kcal**

*Blend all the ingredients into your blender until smooth. Add ice to get the required consistency.

Spinach Cucumber Cool Detox

This smoothie is a little mix of a bunch of different smoothies with minimal ingredients. The smoothie contains spinach, cucumber, and mint, all of which are rich in antioxidants and all vitamins. Together, they improve your overall health and protect you from various diseases. Also, super low in calories!

Ingredients :

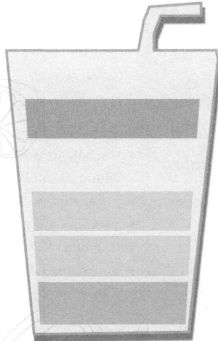

- **1 cup spinach leaves**
- **1/2 lemon**
- **1/2 cucumber**
- **1/2 tsp roasted cumin powder**
- **A handful of mint leaves**

Nutritional :

- Total Fat: 0,4 g
- Sodium: 30 mg
- Carbohydrates: 7,4 g
- Dietary fiber: 2,1 g
- Total sugars: 2,6 g
- Protein : 2,2 g
- Calcium : 74 mg
- Potassium : 434 mg
- Cholesterol : 0 mg

1 cups   *5 mins*   **54 kcal**

*Blend all the ingredients into your blender until smooth. Add ice to get the required consistency.

Purple Power Detox

This smoothie has everything and beyond when you talk about detoxing. It's filled with vitamin C, fiber, vitamin K, manganese, folate, and antioxidants. The add-in flaxseeds and yogurt make this smoothie rich, creamy, filling, and full of fiber.

Ingredients :

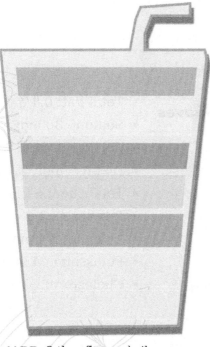

- **½ cup strawberries**
- **Juice of ½ lemon**
- **½ cup curly kale**
- **1 cup apple juice**
- **1 cup frozen blueberries**
- **1 cup regular pear**
- **½ cup yogurt**

!ADD: 2 tbsp flaxseed oil.

Nutritional :

- Total Fat: 15,3 g
- Sodium: 52 mg
- Carbohydrates: 62 g
- Dietary fiber: 4,4 g
- Total sugars: 54,1 g
- Protein : 4,8 g
- Calcium :137 mg
- Potassium : 449 mg
- Cholesterol : 4 mg

 1 cups   **5 mins**   **394 kcal**

*Blend all the ingredients into your blender until smooth.

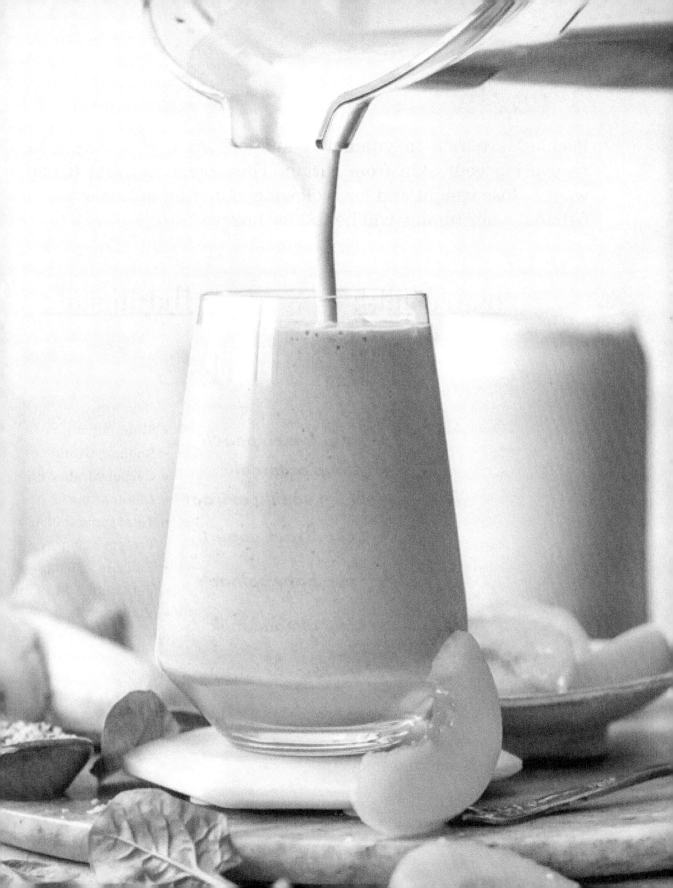

Peaches and Cream Oatmeal

Peaches are rich in vitamin C and collagen, which help in recovering your skin from within. This recipe is great if you want to lose weight and have glowing skin. And because of the oatmeal, your tummy will be full for hours.

Ingredients :

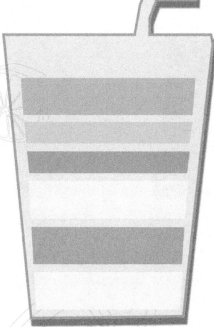

- **1 cup frozen peach**
- **¼ cup oatmeal**
- **¼ tsp vanilla extract**
- **1 cup Greek yogurt**
- **1 cup baby spinach**
- **1 cup almond milk**

Nutritional :

- Total Fat: 4 g
- Sodium: 61 mg
- Carbohydrates: 46 g
- Dietary fiber: 5 g
- Total sugars: 22 g
- Protein : 29 g
- Calcium : 79 mg
- Potassium : 1159 mg
- Cholesterol : 0 mg

1 cups   2 mins   331 kcal

*Blend! Blend! Blend! And enjoy!

Fruity Kale Detox

Have this vitamin and nutrient-dense smoothie regularly to detox as well as strengthen your body against diseases. The calcium, minerals, vitamins, and antioxidants present in this smoothie help support your immune system and cardiovascular health.

Ingredients :

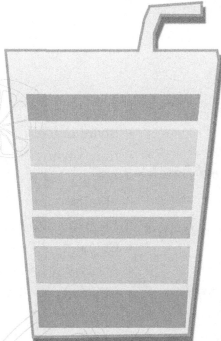

- **4 baby kale leaves**
- **1/2 cup green grapes**
- **a handful of mint leaves**
- **1/2 tsp pepper**
- **1/2 grapefruit**
- **1/2 cup watermelon**

!ADD: a pinch of salt.

Nutritional :

- Total Fat: 0,4 g
- Sodium: 157 mg
- Carbohydrates: 19 g
- Dietary fiber: 1,7 g
- Total sugars: 16,6 g
- Protein : 1,3 g
- Calcium :24 mg
- Potassium : 275 mg
- Cholesterol : 0 mg

 1 cups   **5 mins**   **109 kcal**

*Blend all the ingredients into your blender until smooth.

Watermelon Ginger

This quick **Watermelon Ginger** smoothie is an amazing detoxifier rich in beta-carotene and lycopene. Don't throw away the seeds of the watermelon. They are rich in minerals, zinc, and selenium. The added ginger works as a calorie burner and speeds up the process of weight loss.

Ingredients :

- *1 tsp grated fresh ginger root*
- *1 tbsp chopped fresh mint*
- *Juice of 1 small lime*
- *2 cups watermelon*

Nutritional :

- Total Fat: 0,5 g
- Sodium: 6 mg
- Carbohydrates: 30 g
- Dietary fiber: 3,6 g
- Total sugars: 19,7 g
- Protein : 3 g
- Calcium : 33 mg
- Potassium : 444 mg
- Cholesterol : 0 mg

1 cups   **5 mins**   **115 kcal**

*Blend all the ingredients into your blender until smooth.

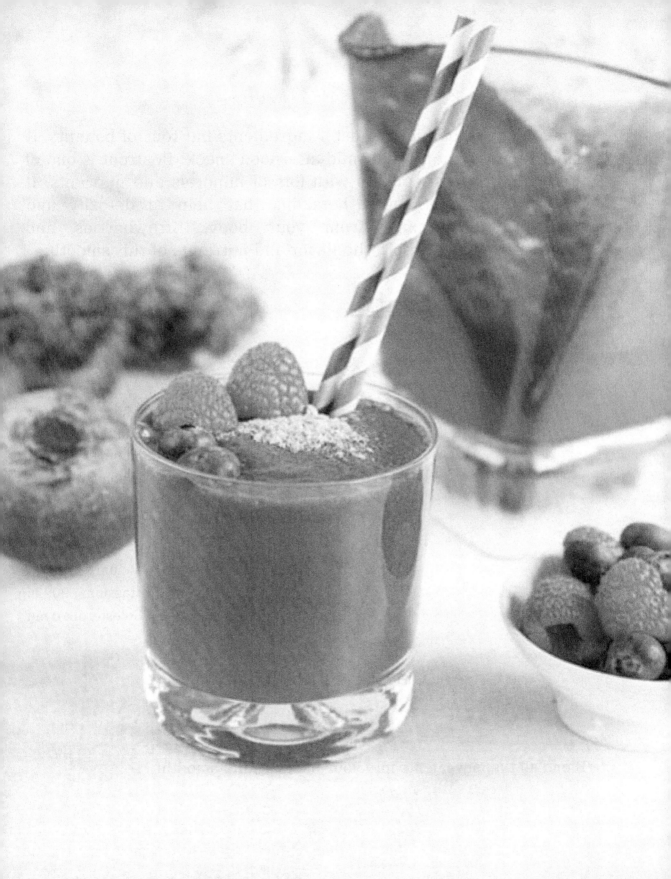

Beet Detox

Beet Detox smoothie has just 4 ingredients but tons of benefits. It is perfect for a morning or mid-afternoon snack. Beetroot is one of the healthiest food sources with lots of minerals and nutrients. It has phytonutrients called betalains that help to detoxify and remove excess toxins from your body. Strawberries and blueberries enhance both the flavor and nutrients of this smoothie.

Ingredients :

- *1 beet small, peeled*
- *1 banana small*
- *1/4 cup blueberries*
- *1 cup strawberries*
- *1-1/2 cup water*

Nutritional :

- Total Fat: 2 g
- Sodium: 1 mg
- Carbohydrates: 85 g
- Dietary fiber: 9 g
- Total sugars: 30 g
- Protein : 6 g
- Calcium : 47 mg
- Potassium : 909 mg
- Cholesterol : 0 mg

!Spetification: Cut beet into half and boil for at least 20-30 minutes.

 1 cups   **5 mins**   **207 kcal**

*Blend all the ingredients into your blender until smooth.

Sunrise Detox

This smoothie is a nourishing breakfast recipe made with frozen bananas, pineapple mangoes, and strawberries. It supports your immune system and heart health and provides you enough energy to go through the day.

Ingredients :

Nutritional :

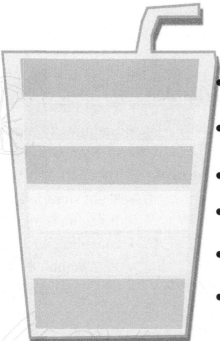

- **½ cup frozen strawberries**
- **1 medium frozen banana**
- **½ cup frozen mango**
- **½ cup pineapple**
- **1 juice of a lemon**
- **1 cup coconut water**

- Total Fat: 2 g
- Sodium: 258 mg
- Carbohydrates: 75 g
- Dietary fiber: 13 g
- Total sugars: 46 g
- Protein : 6 g
- Calcium : 36 mg
- Potassium : 1510 mg
- Cholesterol : 0 mg

1 cups   **5 mins**   **296 kcal**

*Blend! Blend! Blend! Pour into cup and enjoy!

Vegan Detox & Fat Burn

This is a multi-ingredient smoothie in which each ingredient is rich in vitamins, minerals, and tons of antioxidants. Tomatoes lower blood cholesterol levels and protect you from various types of cancer. Carrot and the rest of the ingredients are rich in antioxidants, vitamins A, K, C, fiber, biotin, and minerals. It supports the eye health cardiovascular system.

Ingredients :

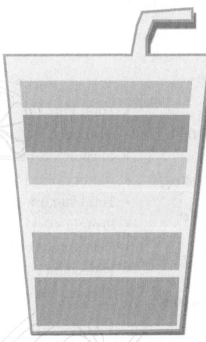

- **A handful of coriander leaves**
- **1 tomato**
- **Freshly ground pepper**
- **1/2 lemon juice**
- **1 celery**
- **1/2 cup baby carrots**

Nutritional :

- Total Fat: 1 g
- Sodium: 85 mg
- Carbohydrates: 75 g
- Dietary fiber: 9 g
- Total sugars: 30 g
- Protein : 6 g
- Calcium : 47 mg
- Potassium : 909 mg
- Cholesterol : 0 mg

!ADD: 1 teaspoon roasted cumin seed powder, salt.

1 cups   **5 mins**   **207 kcal**

*Blend! Blend! Blend! Pour into cup and enjoy!

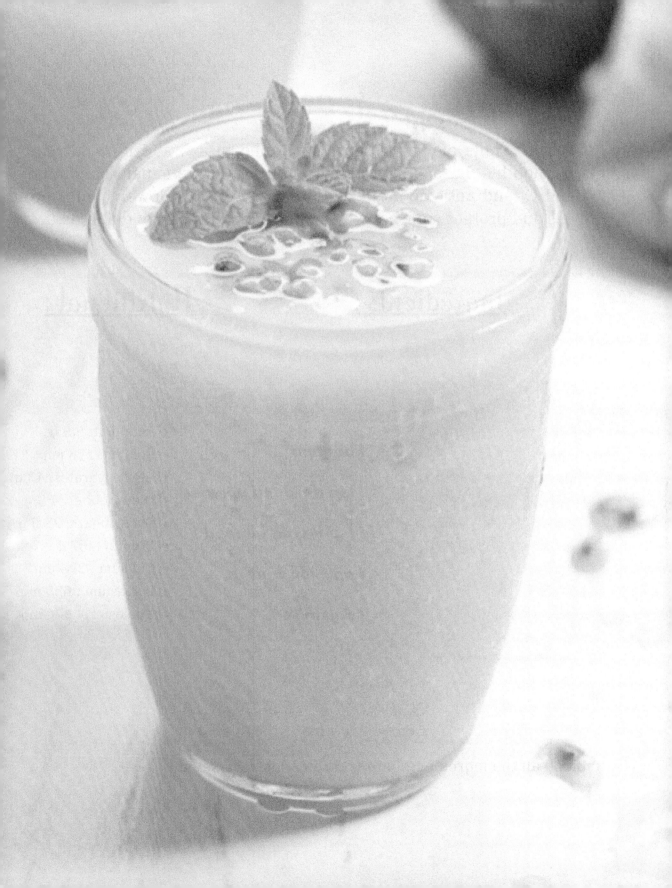

Banana Passion Detox

It is your same old ingredients combined in a brand new nutrient-rich smoothie. Passionfruit is rich in dietary fiber, minerals, vitamins A and C, and antioxidants. Almonds are useful to lower cholesterol levels and protect your body from high blood pressure. diabetes.

Ingredients :

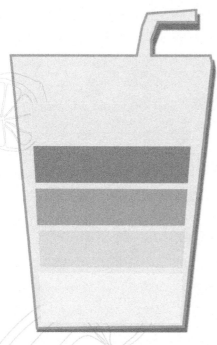

- **1 banana**
- **1 tsp flaxseed powder**
- **1 tsp flaked almond**
- **1 passion fruit**
- **1 cup milk**

Nutritional :

- Total Fat: 5,5 g
- Sodium: 276 mg
- Carbohydrates: 43 g
- Dietary fiber: 4,9 g
- Total sugars: 27,5 g
- Protein : 9,7 g
- Calcium : 298 mg
- Potassium : 625 mg
- Cholesterol : 20 mg

1 cups   **5 mins**   **244 kcal**

*Blend all the ingredients into your blender until smooth.

Spicy Pineapple Detox

This delicious belly-flattening smoothie will help you in getting results much faster. With various ingredients popular for their capacity to detoxify your body, this refreshing Spicy smoothie is the start to a hot-girl (or boy) summer body. This smoothie will help you to your digestion, support eye health, boost your and & immune system, reduce inflammation, and hydrate your body.

Ingredients :

Nutritional :

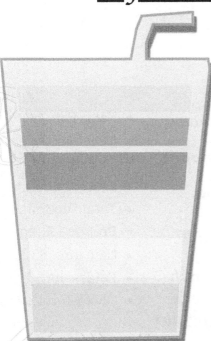

- ½ tsp lime zest
- ½ jalapeno without seeds
- 1 cup cucumber
- 1 tsp lemon juice
- 1 cup fresh or frozen pineapple
- 1 cup coconut water

- Total Fat: 1 g
- Sodium: 83 mg
- Carbohydrates: 76 g
- Dietary fiber: 9 g
- Total sugars: 30 g
- Protein : 6 g
- Calcium : 47 mg
- Potassium : 900 mg
- Cholesterol : 0 mg

1 cups   **3 mins**   **207 kcal**

*Blend all the ingredients into your blender until smooth.

Lime Coconut Green

This is a smoothie you can have as a breakfast replacement. The ingredients are easily available in your house so you make it anytime. The creaminess from the coconut matches perfectly with the tangy lime, creating a match made in heaven. The Greek yogurt added to the smoothie will fill your stomach for longer.

Ingredients :

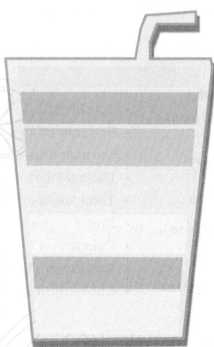

- *juice of 1 lime*
- *1/4 cup mint leaves*
- *1/2 mango, chopped*
- *1 frozen banana*
- *1/2 cup coconut milk*
- *Handful of spinach*
- *1/2 cup Greek yogurt*

Nutritional :

- Total Fat: 29,4 g
- Sodium: 27 mg
- Carbohydrates:33 g
- Dietary fiber: 6,9 g
- Total sugars: 27 g
- Protein : 4,9 g
- Calcium : 83 mg
- Potassium : 702 mg
- Cholesterol : 0 mg

1 cups   **5 mins**   **321 kcal**

*Blend all the ingredients into your blender until smooth.

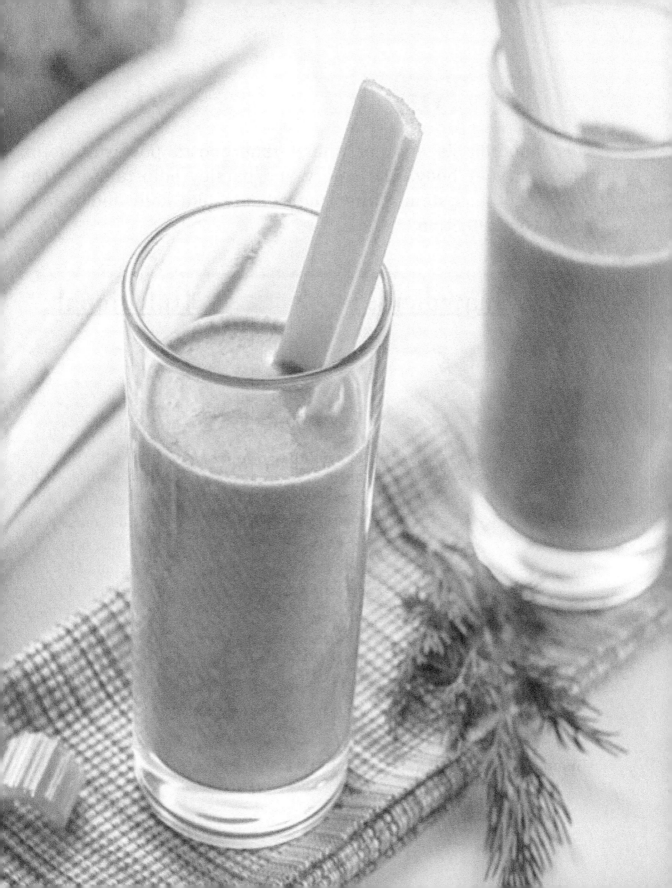

The Super Green Detox

This smoothie is another shake that boosts powerful detox action in your body. The celery and parsley help take out the toxins in the system. Other ingredients like kale and mango boost your nutrition.

Ingredients :

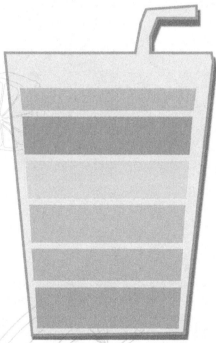

- **1¼ cups cut kale leaves**
- **¼ cup chopped fresh mint**
- **2 medium ribs celery, chopped**
- **¼ cup cut flat-leaf parsley**
- **1¼ cups frozen cubed mango**
- **1 cup chilled fresh orange juice**

Nutritional :

- Total Fat: 1,3 g
- Sodium: 51 mg
- Carbohydrates:58 g
- Dietary fiber: 6,3 g
- Total sugars: 41,5 g
- Protein : 6,1 g
- Calcium : 183 mg
- Potassium :1175 mg
- Cholesterol : 0 mg

2 cups   **15 mins**   **245 kcal**

*Blend! Blend! Blend! Separate into two cups and enjoy!

Berry Breakfast

Berry Breakfast smoothie is easy to make and looks delicious when served. Do not let the beauty of this smoothie fool you. The berries activate the detoxifying enzymes, fiber, and the ginger helps indigestion.

Ingredients :

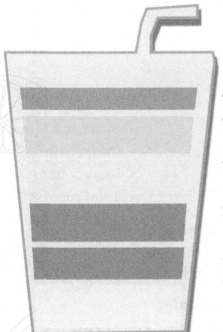

- *1 tsp ground flaxseed*
- *2 tsp grated fresh ginger*
- *1-2 tsp fresh lemon juice*
- *1/4 cup icy pitted cherries*
- *1 cup icy raspberries*
- *3/4 cup chilled almond or rice milk*

Nutritional :

- Total Fat: 1,7 g
- Sodium: 35 mg
- Carbohydrates:33 g
- Dietary fiber: 5,6 g
- Total sugars: 16,5 g
- Protein : 1,5 g
- Calcium : 30 mg
- Potassium : 187 mg
- Cholesterol : 0 mg

2 cups   **5 mins**   **154 kcal**

*Blend all the ingredients into your blender until smooth.

Hail to the Kale Detox

This powerful detox smoothie can be your everyday morning routine as it takes out all the toxins in your body. This can last for more than one day in the fridge. So you can make more than one serving.

Ingredients :

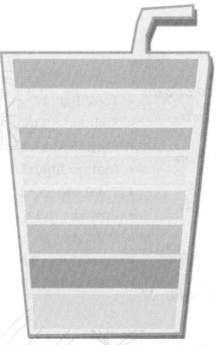

- ½ cucumber
- ½ pear
- ¼ avocado
- ½ lemon
- ½ inch ginger
- handful of cilantro
- 1 cup kale (packed)
- ½ cup coconut water

Nutritional :

- Total Fat: 6,1 g
- Sodium: 121 mg
- Carbohydrates: 19 g
- Dietary fiber: 4,9 g
- Total sugars: 7,3 g
- Protein : 14,1 g
- Calcium : 148 mg
- Potassium :811 mg
- Cholesterol : 32 mg

!ADD: 1 scoop of protein powder (hemp, pumpkin, or pea works great!), if it is too consistent, add water

2 cups　　**5 mins**　　**177kcal**

*Blend all the ingredients into your blender until smooth.

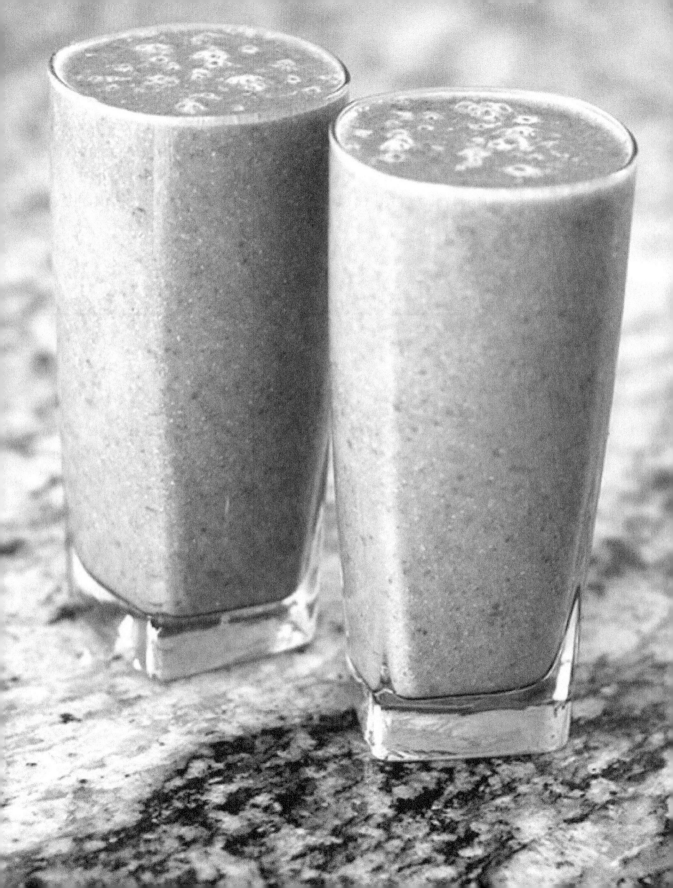

Alkalinity Bliss Detox

Has this wholesome smoothie packed with fiber and other nutritions? This one does not have a weird taste like your other smoothies. Easy to make, this can be your daily nutritional intake.

Ingredients :

- **1 scoop of protein powder**
- **½ pear**
- **¼ avocado**
- **1 packed cup spinach**
- **½ cup almond milk**
- **¼ cup coconut water**

Nutritional :

- Total Fat: 34,6 g
- Sodium: 91 mg
- Carbohydrates: 17 g
- Dietary fiber: 6,1 g
- Total sugars: 8,8 g
- Protein : 15,1 g
- Calcium : 97 mg
- Potassium : 724 mg
- Cholesterol : 32 mg

!ADD: 1 tsp chia seeds, if it is too consistent, add water

 2 cups   **5 mins**   **416 kcal**

*Blend all the ingredients into your blender until smooth.

Sweet Spirit Detox

Do not panic because of its dark color and smell. This smoothie includes spirulina which is a form of microalgae and helps majorly in detoxification. Making this detox smoothie at home is quite easy.

Ingredients :

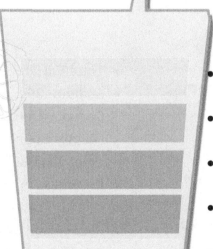

- ½ *banana*
- ¼ *avocado*
- ½ *cup blueberries*
- *1 tsp spirulina*
- ½ *cup almond milk*

Nutritional :

- Total Fat: 19,4 g
- Sodium: 11 mg
- Carbohydrates: 17 g
- Dietary fiber: 4,7 g
- Total sugars: 9,3 g
- Protein : 2,5 g
- Calcium : 14 mg
- Potassium :413 mg
- Cholesterol : 0 mg

!ADD: 1 scoop vanilla protein powder (hemp, pumpkin, or pea works great!), if it is too consistent, add water

2 cups   5 mins   236 kcal

*Blend all the ingredients into your blender until smooth.

Belly Soother Detox

Treat yourself to the delicious and healthy dose of probiotics found in this smoothie. The tangy kefir and papaya satisfy your cravings and give essential nutrients to the body.

Ingredients :

- *1 tbsp raw honey*

- *1 cup papaya*

- *juice from ½ lime*

- *1 cup coconut kefir*

Nutritional :

- Total Fat: 3,3 g
- Sodium: 29 mg
- Carbohydrates: 29 g
- Dietary fiber: 2,3 g
- Total sugars: 25,5 g
- Protein : 1 g
- Calcium : 142 mg
- Potassium : 152 mg
- Cholesterol : 0 mg

!Optional: Coconut kefir you can replace with a coconut yogurt, or cultured coconut milk

2 cups   **5 mins**   **141 kcal**

*Blend all the ingredients into your blender until smooth.

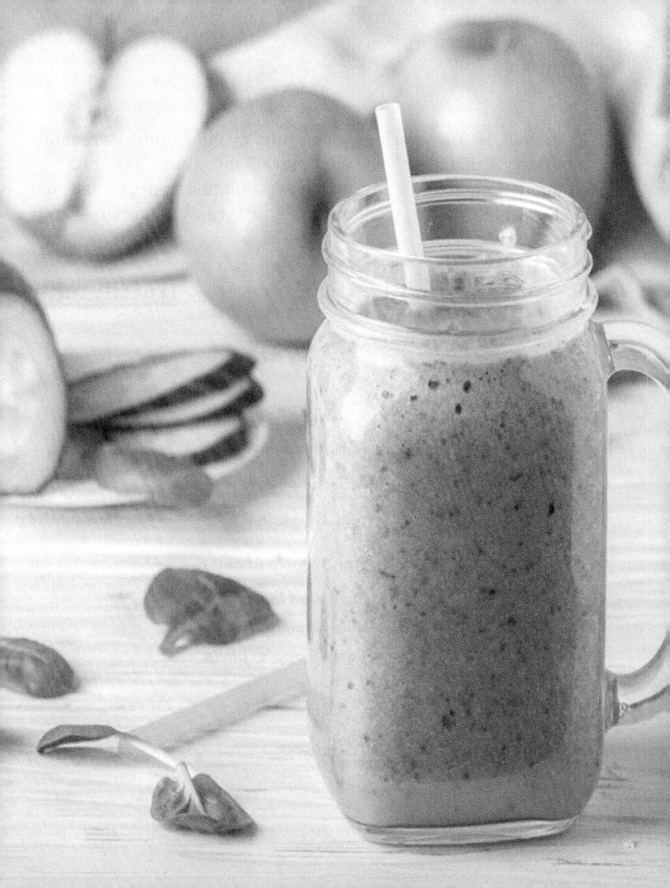

Glorious Morning Detox

Cucumber is the perfect base f0r a mild and refreshing smoothie. Cucumber is the ingredient that has all the nutritions and it replaces major ingredients that you use for health benefits. This smoothie uses a large cucumber as the base.

Ingredients :

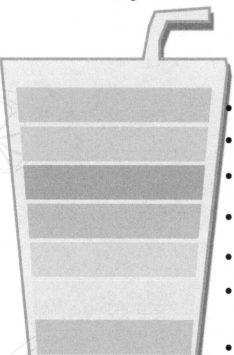

- **A fistful of romaine**
- **1 large cucumber**
- **A fistful of kale**
- **1 big broccoli**
- **2 or 3 stalks of celery**
- **½ peeled lemon, quartered**
- **1 green apple, parts**

!ADD: If it is too consistent, add water

Nutritional :

- Total Fat: 0,6 g
- Sodium: 48 mg
- Carbohydrates: 30 g
- Dietary fiber: 5,8 g
- Total sugars: 15,6 g
- Protein : 4 g
- Calcium : 102 mg
- Potassium : 748 mg
- Cholesterol : 0 mg

 2 cups   **5 mins**   **122 kcal**

*Blend all the ingredients into your blender until smooth.

Smooth Operator Detox

Treat yourself to some smoothie rich in Vitamin C with the detoxifying features of lettuce leaves and cucumber. The other ingredients in this recipe are helpful for your immunity and the perfect choice to intake daily.

Ingredients :

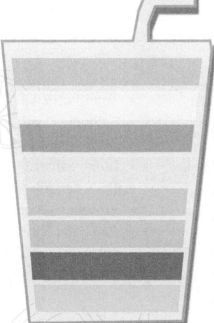

- ¼ avocado,½ apple
- ½ cup jicama
- 5 lettuce leaves
- 1 whole lime
- ½ cucumber
- 4 scoops of hemp protein
- 1 Medjool date
- handful of cilantro

Nutritional :

- Total Fat: 5,4 g
- Sodium: 12 mg
- Carbohydrates: 23 g
- Dietary fiber: 6,1 g
- Total sugars: 11,8 g
- Protein : 2,1 g
- Calcium : 23 mg
- Potassium : 559 mg
- Cholesterol : 0 mg

!ADD: If it is too consistent, add water

2 cups   **5 mins**   **134 kcal**

*Blend all the ingredients into your blender until smooth.

Crazy Sexy Goddess Detox

The avocado and cucumber greens mixed with coconut water will take you on a refreshing journey. This smoothie is the perfect choice for summer days. Plus, it is easy to make at home.

Ingredients :

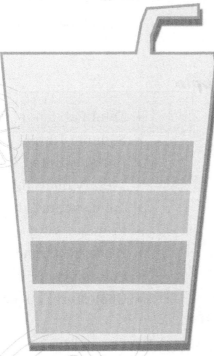

- *1 banana*
- *1 cup blueberries*
- *1 avocado*
- *A fistful of kale or romaine or spinach*
- *1 large cucumber*

Nutritional :

- Total Fat: 20,3 g
- Sodium: 11 mg
- Carbohydrates: 39 g
- Dietary fiber: 11,4 g
- Total sugars: 17,6 g
- Protein : 4,3 g
- Calcium : 51 mg
- Potassium : 1015 mg
- Cholesterol : 0 mg

!ADD: If it is too consistent, add water

 2 cups   **5 mins**   **327 kcal**

*Blend all the ingredients into your blender until smooth.

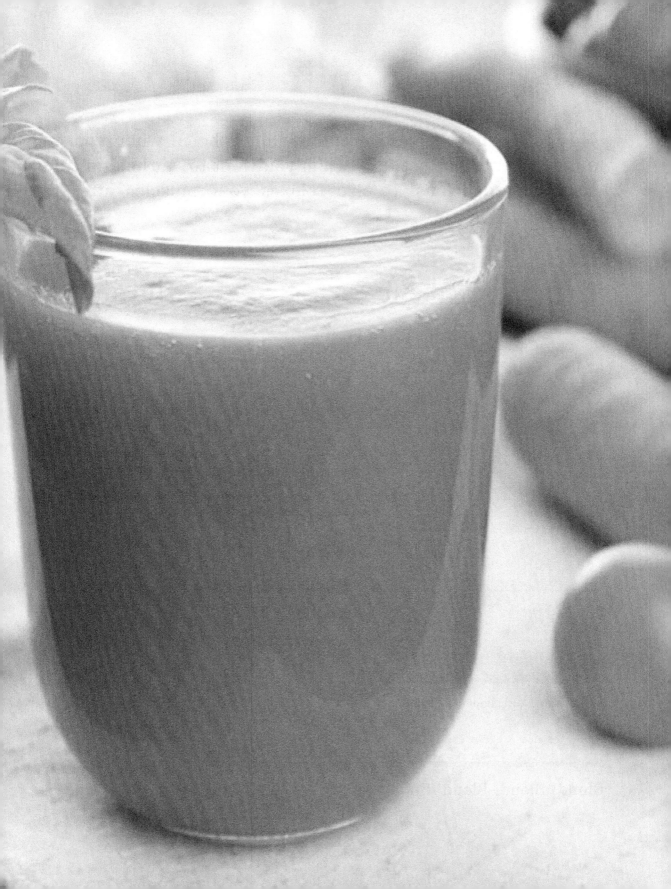

The Sicilian Detox

This refreshing, spicy drink is a filling choice when you feel hungry. It is a perfect take when you want to eat healthily and something delicious. It also relaxes your muscles after the workout.

Ingredients :

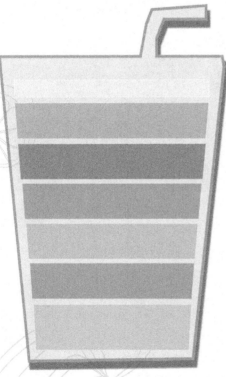

- **4 cloves garlic**
- **6 carrots**
- **2 red bell peppers**
- **3 large tomatoes**
- **4 stalks celery**
- **1 cup loosely packed spinach**
- **1 cup watercress**

!**Optional:** 1 red jalapeño, seeded.

Nutritional :

- Total Fat: 1,1 g
- Sodium: 185 mg
- Carbohydrates: 41 g
- Dietary fiber: 10,4 g
- Total sugars: 22,8 g
- Protein : 6,4 g
- Calcium : 132 mg
- Potassium : 1628 mg
- Cholesterol : 0 mg

 2 cups   **5 mins**   **181 kcal**

*Blend! Blend! Blend! Separate into two cups and enjoy!

Strawberry Fields Detox

Berries are also great for detoxifying your body. Strawberries supply a bounty of anti-inflammatory and antioxidants due to phytonutrient factories.

Ingredients :

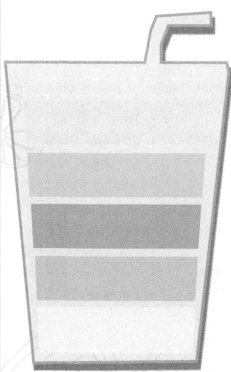

- **1 tbsp lemon zest**
- **1 banana**
- **2 cups fresh strawberries**
- **1½ cups loosely packed spinach**
- **1 small orange**
- **3 cups cashew or nondairy milk**

Nutritional :

- Total Fat: 20,3 g
- Sodium: 11 mg
- Carbohydrates: 39 g
- Dietary fiber: 11,4 g
- Total sugars: 17,6 g
- Protein : 4,3 g
- Calcium : 51 mg
- Potassium : 1015 mg
- Cholesterol : 0 mg

 2 cups   **5 mins**   **532 kcal**

*Blend all the ingredients into your blender until smooth.

Lemon Blueberry Detox

Make this smoothie that's vegan, sugar-free, and guilt-free but utterly delicious. This super simple recipe is all you need for energy-boosting and to fill an empty stomach.

Ingredients :

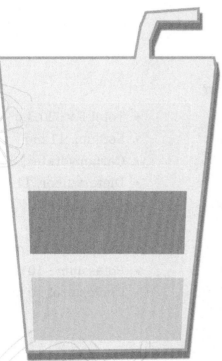

- *1 organic lemon (whole).*
- *¼ cup organic blueberries*
- *1 cup alkaline water*

Nutritional :

- Total Fat: 0,2 g
- Sodium: 1 mg
- Carbohydrates: 5,3 g
- Dietary fiber: 1,3 g
- Total sugars: 2,5 g
- Protein : 0,5 g
- Calcium : 8 mg
- Potassium : 54 mg
- Cholesterol : 0 mg

 3 cups   **5 mins**   **191 kcal**

*Blend all the ingredients into your blender until smooth.

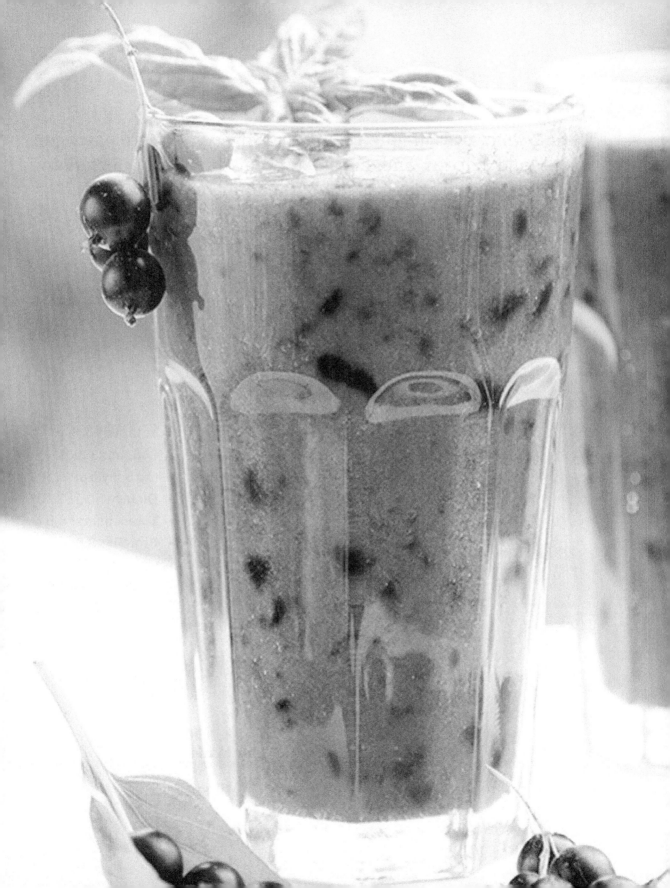

Mint Apple Berry Detox

TIt is a simple yet unique recipe that gives you the pleasure of apples and berries and boosts protein. It is a perfect detox recipe that would take less than 5 minutes to prepare.

Ingredients :

Nutritional :

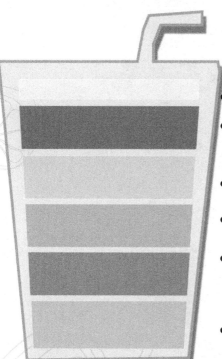

- **2 tbsp of Hemp Hearts**
- **3-4 leaves of green leaf lettuce**
- **½ green apple**
- **8 mint leaves**
- **¼ cup fresh /frozen berry**
- **8-12 oz pure water**

- Total Fat: 4,5 g
- Sodium: 3 mg
- Carbohydrates: 9,3 g
- Dietary fiber: 2,7 g
- Total sugars: 5,9 g
- Protein : 3,9 g
- Calcium : 15 mg
- Potassium : 898 mg
- Cholesterol : 0 mg

 2 cups   5 mins   90 kcal

*Blend all the ingredients into your blender until smooth.

Blueberry Ginger Detox

This is a gluten-free smoothie that is packed with antioxidants. With just four ingredients, this can fill your hunger along with beneficial nutrients. The ingredients are easily available.

Ingredients :

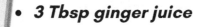

- **3 Tbsp ginger juice**

- **1 frozen banana**

- **¼ cup blueberries**

- **1 cup milk of choice**

Nutritional :

- Total Fat: 29,3 g
- Sodium: 21 mg
- Carbohydrates: 28 g
- Dietary fiber: 28,5 g
- Total sugars: 5,6 g
- Protein : 4,3 g
- Calcium : 32mg
- Potassium : 650 mg
- Cholesterol : 0 mg

2 cups   **5 mins**   **367 kcal**

*Blend all the ingredients into your blender until smooth.

Detox Smoothies for Our Heart and Liver

Taking care of your heart and liver is one the most important things you can do for your health and eating right, including lots of fiber, is the best way to do it. Eating fast food, high in carbs and unhealthy fats leads to high cholesterol, which can affect the heart. Moreover, if your diet contains high amounts of cholesterol, then the fat can build up on your liver, ultimately leading to liver failure and other problems. Scary right? However, if you eat right, you can prevent it from happening, and there is no better alternative than combining all the nutrient-rich ingredients into a smoothie! Smoothies, when made with the right ingredients in the right amounts, can fulfill your daily intake of cholesterol-reducing fiber, tons of antioxidants, and omega-3's which support your heart health. Many food items can improve your heart and liver health such as berries, nuts, spices, and dark green vegetables. Toss them into a blender and you have got yourself a smoothie packed full of nutrients. Here are some of my favorite heart and liver detox smoothie recipes you can make any time.

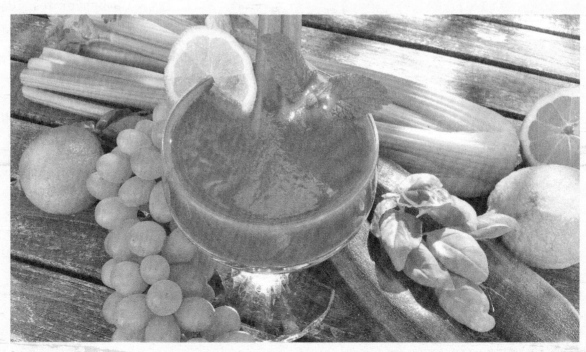

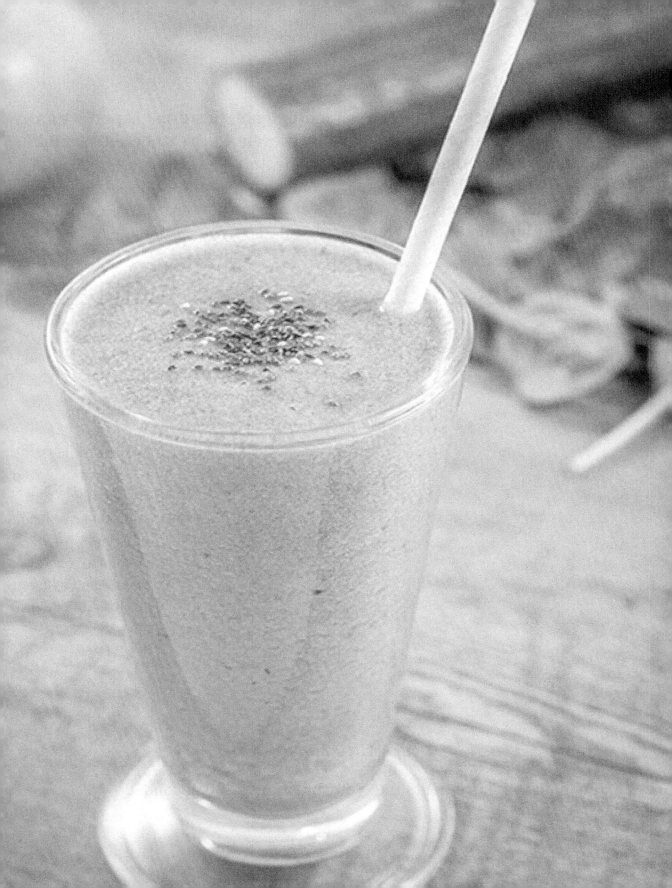

Green Lemonade

Packed with delicious and fresh ingredients, this drink is perfect for summer. The apples and cucumber present in the smoothie are full of antioxidants that help reduce cholesterol levels. The lemon and spinach are full of vitamins, iron, magnesium, folic acid, acid potassium, B-complex vitamins, and many more nutrients and prevent inflammation in your body and keep your organs healthy.

Ingredients :

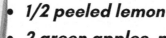

- 1/2 peeled lemon
- 2 green apples peeled and seeds
- 1 cup baby spinach
- ½ peeled cucumber
- 3/4 cup of water
- 4-5 ice cubes

Nutritional :

- Total Fat: 1,3 g
- Sodium: 37 mg
- Carbohydrates: 73 g
- Dietary fiber: 13,8 g
- Total sugars: 50,5 g
- Protein : 3,7 g
- Calcium : 76 mg
- Potassium : 948 mg
- Cholesterol : 0 mg

1 cups   **10 mins**   **278 kcal**

*Blend all the ingredients into your blender for 30 second.

Blueberry Avocado

Blueberries contain a lot of antioxidants and phytochemicals and avocados have monounsaturated fatty acids. Blended, they help in lowering the risk of heart problems. Avocados also contain folic acid and vitamin B6, which are great for a healthy heart.

Ingredients :

- **One protein powder**
- **1 cup blueberries**
- **1/4 avocado**
- **Juice of 1/2 lime**
- **1 cup coconut water**
- **4 ice cubes**

Nutritional :

- Total Fat: 10,3 g
- Sodium: 4 mg
- Carbohydrates: 25 g
- Dietary fiber: 6,9 g
- Total sugars: 14,7 g
- Protein : 32,1 g
- Calcium : 7 mg
- Potassium : 355 mg
- Cholesterol : 0 mg

! Swetened to taste (honey, stevia, etc.)

1 cups   **5 mins**   **186 kcal**

*Blend them until you get a smooth and creamy texture. Enjoy!

Green Machine

If you are not a big fan of blending chunks of fruits and veggies, thisprevent this, is the perfect recipe. Both spinach and broccoli sprouts used in the smoothie contain vitamin - B complex, which supports liver health and helps in breaking down fat. Spinach blends quite quickly and smoothly, and broccoli sprouts add a lot of nutrients without affecting the flavor.

Ingredients :

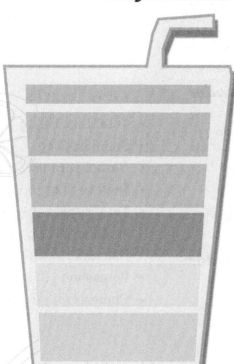

- **2 tbsp nuts or seeds**
- **A handful of baby spinach**
- **½ handful broccoli**
- **1 handful lettuce**
- **2 bananas**
- **4 ice cubes/ water**

Nutritional :

- Total Fat: 9,6 g
- Sodium: 159 mg
- Carbohydrates: 64 g
- Dietary fiber: 9,2 g
- Total sugars: 32,7 g
- Protein : 6 g
- Calcium : 44 mg
- Potassium : 1142 mg
- Cholesterol : 0 mg

 1 cups   **10 mins**   **337 kcal**

*Put all of the ingredients together in a blender and blend until smooth.

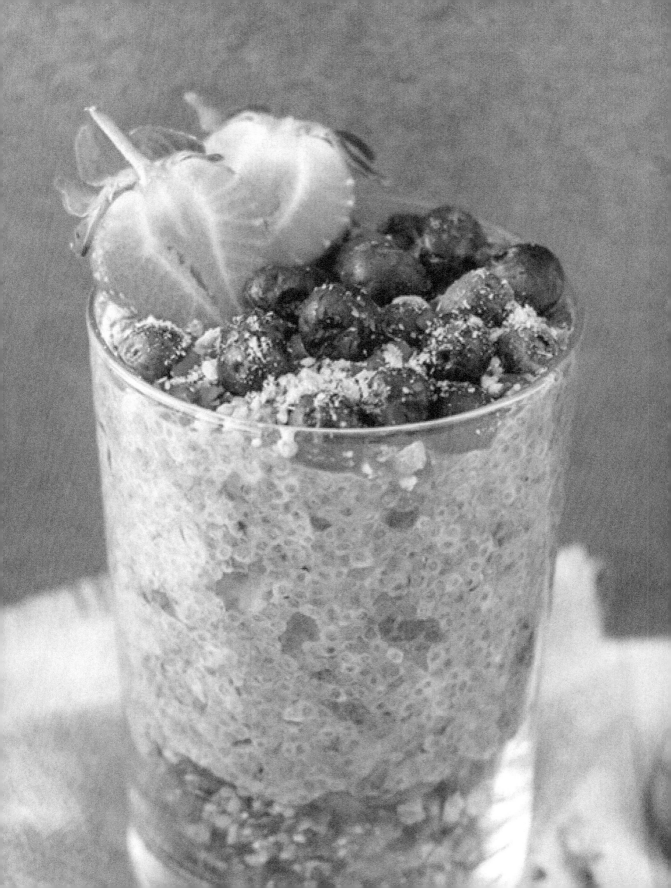

Chia-Seed

Acai berries are high in antioxidants and also increase good cholesterol in your body. Chia seeds, which are also high in antioxidants and omega-3 fatty acids, support cardiovascular health. This low-calorie smoothie is great if you are busy and don't have time for preparation.

Ingredients :

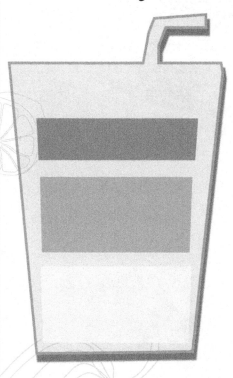

- **3 1/2 oz frozen acai berries**

- **1 – 2 tbsp chia seeds**

- **2 cups unsweet almond milk**

Nutritional :

- Total Fat: 7 g
- Sodium: 360 mg
- Carbohydrates: 4 g
- Dietary fiber: 2 g
- Total sugars: 0 g
- Protein : 2 g
- Calcium : 600 mg
- Potassium : 380 mg
- Cholesterol : 0 mg

! Swetened to taste (honey, stevia, etc.) of you choice.

1 cups   **5 mins**   **80 kcal**

*Blend them until you get a smooth and creamy texture. Enjoy!

Kale Parsley

Parsley acts as an amazing support system for the liver. A high amount of Vitamin C is great for flushing out toxins. Parsley also helps in stimulating bile, which helps break down fats to use as energy. Kale contains vitamins, minerals, omega-3, and many more nutrients that help in preventing the body from chronic illness, blood clotting, fiber and encouraging bone buildup.

Ingredients :

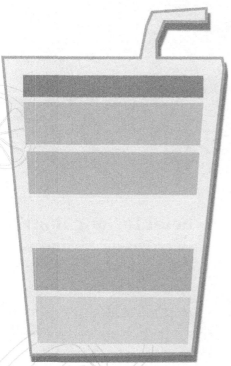

- **4 kale leaves**
- **⅓ bunch parsley**
- **2 chopped celery ribs**
- **Juice of ½ lemon**
- **1 apple wedges**
- **2 cups water**

Nutritional :

- Total Fat: 0,4 g
- Sodium: 61 mg
- Carbohydrates: 62 g
- Dietary fiber: 6,9 g
- Total sugars: 41,2 g
- Protein : 6,6 g
- Calcium : 75 mg
- Potassium : 243 mg
- Cholesterol : 0 mg

 1 cups   **10 mins**   **236 kcal**

*Put all in the blender and blend until you have a smooth consistency. Add in some water if you like and some honey for sweetness.

Chapter 5
Antioxidant-Rich Smoothie Recipes

You may have already noticed by now that ingredients rich in antioxidants are good for your body. But what exactly are antioxidants and how do they benefit our body? We will cover all of that and more in this chapter. Along with that, you will get some delicious antioxidant smoothie recipes that you can prepare with simple ingredients available in your home.

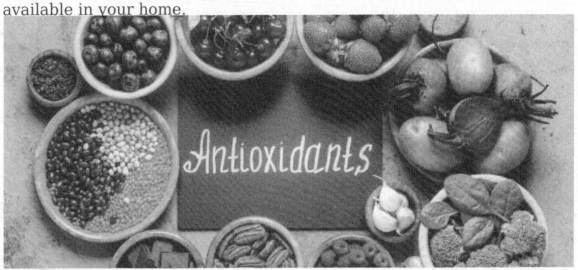

What Are Antioxidants, Why Are They Crucial for our Body?

To understand antioxidants, we need to reference basic science (I promise I will try to make it interesting). We know that atoms contain protons, electrons, and neutrons, and two or more atoms combine to make up a molecule. Now, for the molecule to be stable, it should contain the right number of electrons, or else, it becomes a "free radical". Free radicals act as bad molecules that damage the cells of the body by attacking good molecules. It results in oxidative stress that can cause various diseases like Alzheimer's, cardiovascular diseases, diabetes, Parkinson's disease, and eye diseases. Your body gets exposed to free radicals through sources such as chemicals, smoke, and air pollution. Antioxidants work as the counter attackers that prevent the dangerous free radicals from damaging body cells.

Free radicals are not all bad. They help to fight pathogens that lead to infections in your body. But it is essential to have a balance of antioxidants and free radicals; otherwise, it could damage the DNA and increase the risk of diseases. Although your body produces antioxidants to fight the excess amount of free radicals, the antioxidants present in external sources such as fruits, vegetables, and whole foods help make the process more effective. A study shows that antioxidants act as "radical scavengers, hydrogen donor, electron donor, peroxide decomposer, singlet oxygen quencher, enzyme inhibitor, synergist, and metal-chelating agents" (Lobo et al., 2010). Antioxidants are also proven to increase the shelf life of food sources and are therefore utilized as food preservatives.

Types of Antioxidants and Their Benefits

There are different types of antioxidants and each one has a crucial role in maintaining your health.

- **Phytonutrients**

Phytonutrients or phytochemicals are typically found in plants and have a lot of benefits for your body, one of which is the accessibility of antioxidants. There are over 4000 phytonutrients in the world, but only a few have been studied. Some of them are resveratrol, anthocyanin, lycopene, is flavones, and lutein. These antioxidants mainly support heart health and prevent your body from diseases like cancer.

- **Vitamin E**

Vitamin E is found in eight chemical forms, but the form suitable for human needs is alpha-tocopherol. Apart from helping in the body's normal functioning, this vitamin also controls the number of free radicals in your body. Vitamin E is also good for your skin, reducing inflammation, and eye health!

- **Vitamin A**

The precursors of vitamin A, including alpha-carotene, beta-carotene, and beta-kryptoxanthin, have various antioxidant properties. Although vitamin A is mainly associated with eye health, these precursors help prevent your body from diseases like lung cancer, heart problems, and diabetes.

- **Vitamin C**

The precursor of vitamin C is known as ascorbic acid and is found in many plant-based foods. Apart from playing its role in good immune function, this antioxidant also protects other antioxidants such as vitamin E from the attack of free radicals.

- **Selenium**

Selenium is present in both organic and inorganic types of meat. It can be obtained from both plants and animals. It is a strong antioxidant that prevents your body from cancer and various heart diseases.

- **Manganese**

Manganese is a powerful antioxidant found in the form of an enzyme in your body's mitochondria. And we all know that mitochondria are the "powerhouse of the cell". This antioxidant produces the energy required by your body to function properly.

- **Iron**

Iron is one of the most important antioxidant sources required by the body. It is found in two forms—with protein (heme) and without protein (nonheme). While plant-based foods are rich in nonheme, animal-based food sources are rich in both heme and nonheme iron. Iron protects the cell membrane from getting damaged or oxidized.

- **Copper**

Copper contains an antioxidant and a protein called ceruloplasmin, which helps in transporting iron to the tissues. Although required in small amounts, a lack of copper can affect the level of all the other antioxidants. Copper also works as a pro-oxidant responsible for free-radical damage and lipid oxidation.

Foods Rich in Antioxidants

To work properly, your body must receive essential antioxidants. You can get them by including the following food sources in your diet:

- **Dark Chocolate**

Really? Dark chocolate? That is what most people first think when they learn that dark chocolate is nutritious. But, it is true. Dark chocolate contains more cocoa than regular chocolate and is therefore rich in antioxidants and minerals. The cocoa present in dark chocolate helps to reduce inflammation in the body and lessen the risk of heart diseases. The more cocoa the chocolate has, the more beneficial it is for the body. You can eat a piece or two of dark chocolate to get the required antioxidants in your daily diet.

- **Berries**

Berries of any kind are super-rich in antioxidants. The most commonly used berries are blueberries, strawberries, and raspberries.

● Blueberries are low-calorie food sources that contain the most amount of antioxidants among all fruits and veggies. They delay the weakening of the brain due to age factors.

● Strawberries are the most popular and versatile berries. They are rich in vitamin C and antioxidants that help reduce bad cholesterol levels.

● Raspberries are tart berries used in various desserts and smoothies. Apart from being a great source of antioxidants, they are also rich in vitamin C, dietary fiber, and manganese. The antioxidants in raspberries may help reduce oxidative stress and inflammation.

- **Spinach**

Spinach is one of the vegetables that is packed with tons of nutrients. It's insanely low in calories and is rich in minerals, vitamins, and antioxidants. The antioxidants present in spinach protect your eyes from harmful wavelengths and UV rays. You can include them in any smoothie you want to make it a little more nutritious.

- **Kale**

Kale is another nutritious green vegetable. It is a part of the same vegetable group as cauliflower and broccoli. It contains vitamin A, K, and C, calcium, and other antioxidants that support cellular functioning and bone health.

There are various other amazing sources of antioxidants such as artichokes, beetroots, pomegranate, oranges, nuts and seeds, and carrots. You can combine these ingredients and make yourself a delicious smoothie every day. Don't know how? Use the recipes mentioned in the next section to create your daily dose of antioxidants.

Antioxidant Smoothie Recipes.

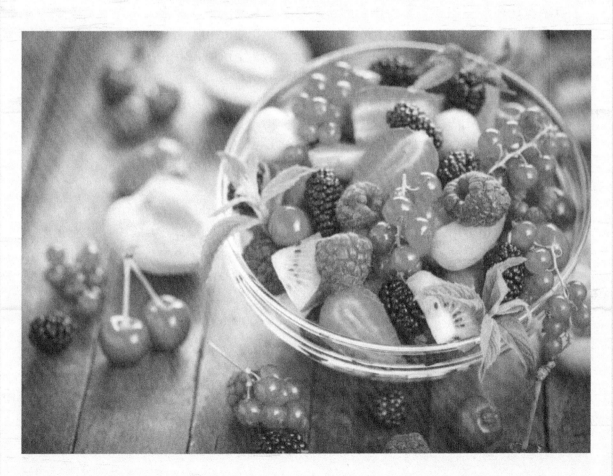

Peanut Butter&Jelly Protein

You will love this smoothie as it has a touch of childishness. This is perfectly fit for post-workout intake and packed with nutrition and protein. It is healthy, and at the same time, tastier than your regular protein diet.

Ingredients :

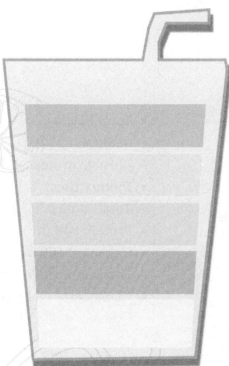

- **1 cup mixed frozen berries**
- **1/4 cup vanilla protein powder**
- **2 tbsp rolled oats**
- **1-2 tbsp of peanut butter**
- **1 cup milk**

Nutritional :

- Total Fat: 11 g
- Sodium: 20 mg
- Carbohydrates: 41 g
- Dietary fiber: 13 g
- Total sugars: 27 g
- Protein : 41 g
- Calcium : 295 mg
- Potassium : 353 mg
- Cholesterol : 20 mg

 1 cups   **5 mins**   **417 kcal**

*Blend all the ingredients into your blender until smooth.

Key Lime Pie Shake

What's better than having a smoothie which is just like a delicious cheat day snack? This mouth-watering shake is low in sugar intake but high in protein. And it can become your new way to have protein but in a tastier way.

Ingredients :

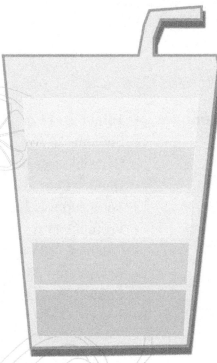

- 1/2 cup Cottage cheese
- 1 scoop protein powder
- 1 tbsp Lime juice
- 1 cup Ice cubes
- 1/2 cup Water

Nutritional :

- Total Fat: 4 g
- Sodium: 527 mg
- Carbohydrates: 17 g
- Dietary fiber: 4,3 g
- Total sugars: 1,3 g
- Protein : 42 g
- Calcium : 189 mg
- Potassium : 287 mg
- Cholesterol : 34 mg

! Optional: add almond milk

1 cups   **5 mins**   **180 kcal**

*Blend all the ingredients into your blender until smooth.

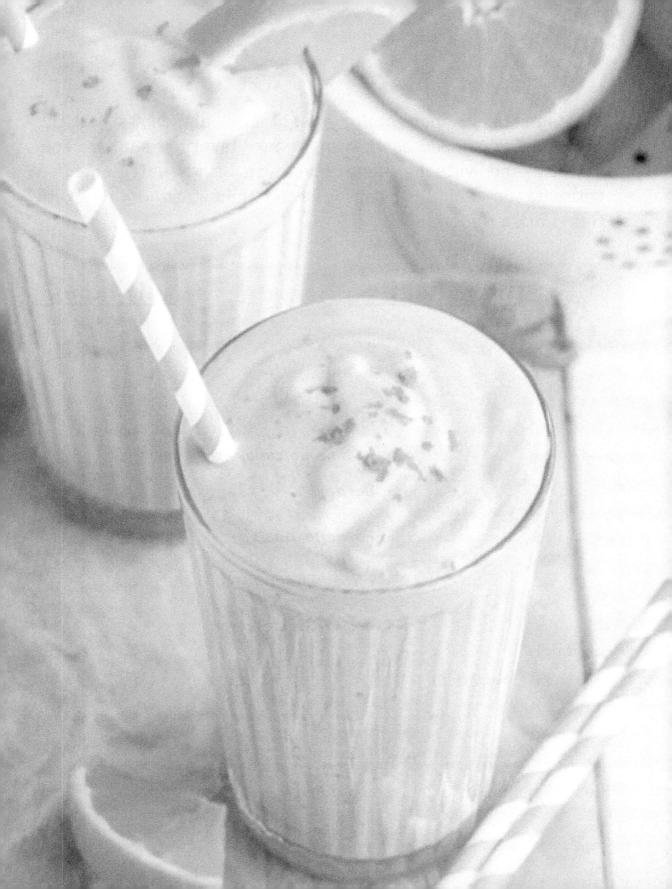

Orange Banana

This smoothie is perfect for weight loss, andwhat's and the taste is as good as having your favorite shake. This smoothieAnd with the name, gives you brings nutrition filled with vitamin c. Nothing can be better than starting a day with this sunrise smoothie.

Ingredients :

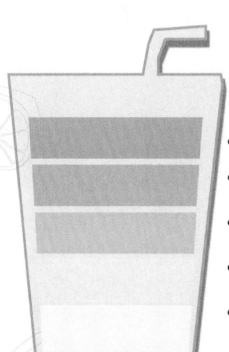

- **1 Cinnamon stick**

- **Berries**

- **1 orange, peeled**

- **1 frozen banana**

- **4-6 oz Greek Yogurt**

Nutritional :

- Total Fat: 1 g
- Sodium: 37 mg
- Carbohydrates: 42 g
- Dietary fiber: 14 g
- Total sugars: 28 g
- Protein : 15 g
- Calcium : 24 mg
- Potassium : 312 mg
- Cholesterol : 20 mg

1 cups   **5 mins**   **350 kcal**

*Blend them until you get a smooth and creamy texture. Enjoy!

Dark Chocolate Peppermint

The shake filled with mint and sweet taste is another perfect way to lose weight. What's better than having chocolate and losing weight at the same time. This smoothie feels like a dessert in your mouth.

Ingredients :

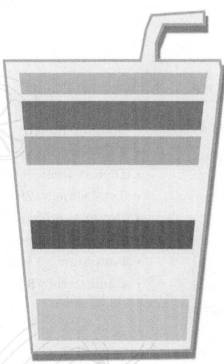

- **1/4 tsp peppermint extract**
- **1 scoop chocolate protein powder**
- **2 tbsp cocoa powder**
- **1 large banana, icy**
- **1 tbsp dark/vegan chocolate chips**
- **1 cup non-fat milk**
- **2-3 large ice cubes**

Nutritional :

- Total Fat: 6 g
- Sodium: 321 mg
- Carbohydrates: 49 g
- Dietary fiber: 11 g
- Total sugars: 24 g
- Protein : 22 g
- Calcium : 24 mg
- Potassium : 521 mg
- Cholesterol : 0 mg

! Topping: homemade whipping cream, vegan whipped topping, or Greek yogurt

1 cups   5 mins   296 kcal

*Blend them until you get a smooth and creamy texture. Enjoy!

The Antioxidant Breakfast

The best antioxidant smoothie for maintaining a healthier life. It helps in the increase in hormones, makes the skin healthier, and slows down early aging. The raw cacao and matcha are rich in providing all the nutrition you require for weight loss and a healthy body. The ingredients are a bit more in this one, but the taste makes it all worth it.

Ingredients :

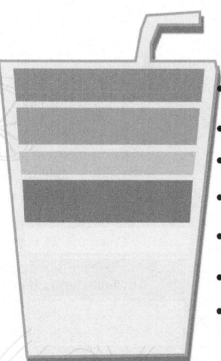

- *1 cup blueberries + 3 strawberries*
- *1 pomegranate (seeds)*
- *1 tbsp rolled oats*
- *½ beetroot*
- *1 tbsp coconut oil*
- *1 lime juice*
- *½ cup natural yogurt*

Nutritional :

- Total Fat: 6,79 g
- Sodium: 50 mg
- Carbohydrates: 40 g
- Dietary fiber: 9,6 g
- Total sugars: 29 g
- Protein : 6,55 g
- Calcium : 11 mg
- Potassium : 334 mg
- Cholesterol : 8 mg

! **Add:** 1 tbsp raw cacao powder, 1 tbsp maca powder

1 cups   **5 mins**   **248 kcal**

*Blend all the ingredients into your blender until smooth.

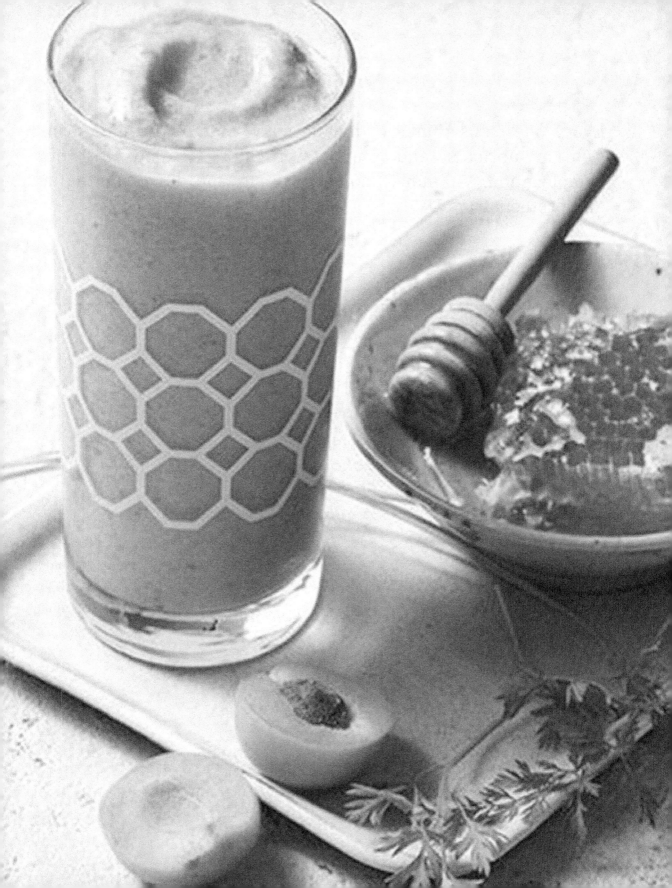

Silky Skin Smoothie

Every one of us thinks of having silky, shiny skin. This drink rich in apricots and carrots provides a glow to your complexation. Vitamin C can help in slowing down skin aging and protects from UV rays.

Ingredients :

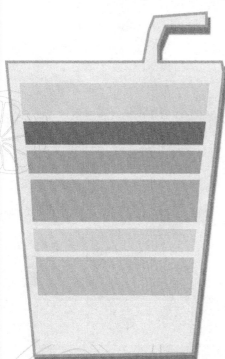

- **1 fresh apricot**
- **1/2 tsp cinnamon**
- **2 chopped dried apricots**
- **¼ cup grated carrot**
- **1 tbsp of honey**
- **½ cup ice cubes**
- **½ cup whole milk yogurt**

Nutritional :

- Total Fat: 3,5 g
- Sodium: 23 mg
- Carbohydrates: 21 g
- Dietary fiber: 3 g
- Total sugars: 17 g
- Protein : 8 g
- Calcium : 65 mg
- Potassium : 467 mg
- Cholesterol : 0 mg

 1 cups   **5 mins**   **130 kcal**

*Blend all the ingredients into your blender until smooth.

Antioxidant Triple- Berry

This smoothie having antioxidant, protein, fiber is the best fit for the healthy and packed breakfast you wish to have. The taste of berries berry with yogurt, flaxseed meal, almond butter, and many other ingredients provide you an extra protective prevention layer from skin-aging, pollution, and many more.

Ingredients :

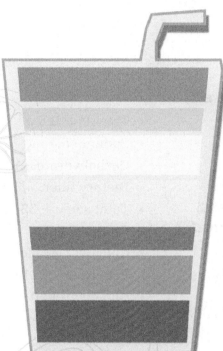

- **2 cups spinach**
- **1 tbsp almond butter**
- **½ cup almond milk**
- **½ cup plain greek yogurt**
- **½ cup raspberries**
- **1/4 cup blueberries**
- **½ cup blackberries**

Nutritional :

- Total Fat: 12,2 g
- Sodium: 50 mg
- Carbohydrates: 57 g
- Dietary fiber: 16,8 g
- Total sugars: 28,4 g
- Protein : 20,1 g
- Calcium : 32 mg
- Potassium : 465 mg
- Cholesterol : 0 mg

! **Add:** 1 tbsp flaxseed meal.

 1 cups   5 mins   391 kcal

*Blend all the ingredients into your blender until smooth.

Cucumber and Apple Winter

For a healthier diet plan during the winters (or anytime), kick start with this sweet and healthy smoothie. This will provide you immunity and boost all day. Cucumbers are rich in antioxidants that will help preserve your skin, reduce inflammation, and help in digesting issues.

Ingredients :

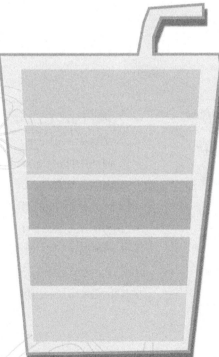

- *1 cucumber, pared and chopped.*
- *1 cup of cubed, frozen mango*
- *2 medium-apples, core removed and cubed.*
- *1 orange, peeled*
- *water to fill line*

Nutritional :

- Total Fat: 0,6 g
- Sodium: 5,4 mg
- Carbohydrates: 13 g
- Dietary fiber: 6,8 g
- Total sugars: 33,7 g
- Protein : 1,7 g
- Calcium : 24 mg
- Potassium : 221 mg
- Cholesterol : 0 mg

1 cups   ***5 mins***   ***164 kcal***

*Blend them until you get a smooth and creamy texture. Enjoy!

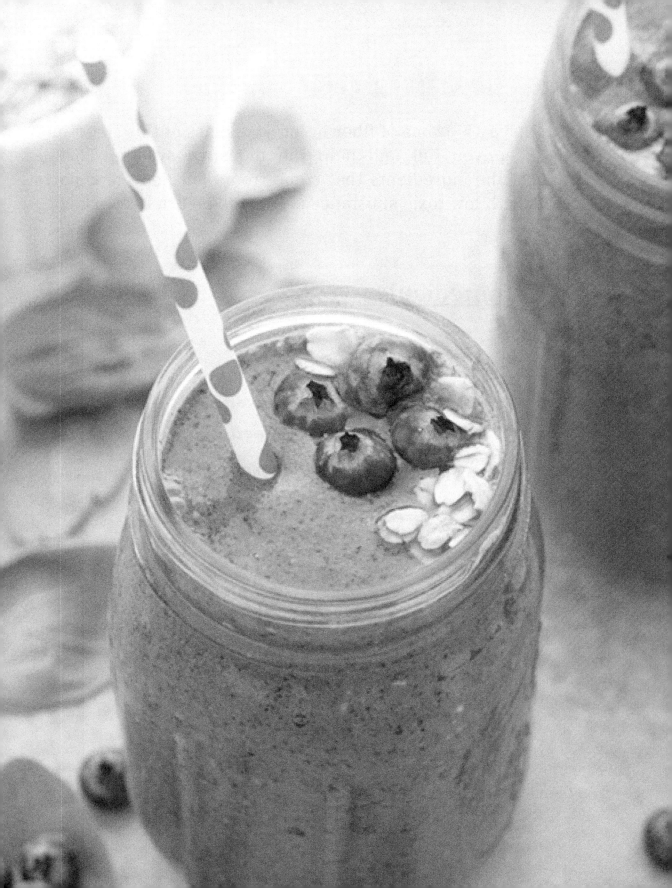

Oats and Berry

You can have 15 grams of fiber in just one glass of this smoothie! It will keep you full and help the digestive system. This is because of the ingredients that come from plant leaves or parts of plants with low toxic substances. This recipe is a keeper!

Ingredients :

- 1/2 cup cooked oats
- 2 tbsp flaxeed
- 1/2 medium apple
- 1 cup spinach
- 1/3 cup blackberries
- 1/3 cup raspberries
- 8 oz almond milk

Nutritional :

- Total Fat: 10 g
- Sodium: 229 mg
- Carbohydrates: 42 g
- Dietary fiber: 15,2 g
- Total sugars: 12 g
- Protein : 9,5 g
- Calcium : 12 mg
- Potassium : 471 mg
- Cholesterol : 0 mg

 1 cups   **5 mins**   **277 kcal**

*In a blender, combine all of the ingredients and blend until smooth.

Vitamin C Antioxidant Pink

This unique vitamin C pink smoothie can be used for breakfast and will provide antioxidant agents to cure your body. From making your day better to protecting your organs, cells from oxidation, this smoothie is best for you.

Ingredients :

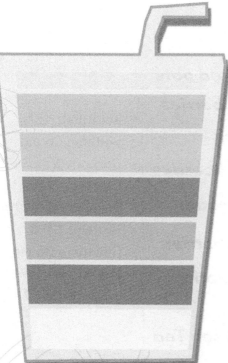

- **1 tsp lemon juice**
- **1 apple, sliced**
- **1 stick celery**
- **1/4 of an avocado**
- **1 cup strawberries**
- **1 piece beet**
- **Almond milk**

Nutritional :

- Total Fat: 12 g
- Sodium: 266 mg
- Carbohydrates: 39 g
- Dietary fiber: 15 g
- Total sugars: 32 g
- Protein : 5 g
- Calcium : 23 mg
- Potassium : 689 mg
- Cholesterol : 0 mg

 1 cups   **5 mins**   **308 kcal**

*Blend all the ingredients into your blender until smooth.

Cleansing Smoothie

The rich ingredient smoothie detoxifies the entire body. The avocado, which is rich in antioxidants and fiber, helps clean your body and improve digestion. And the best part is that you can have any time of the day to cleanse your body.

Ingredients :

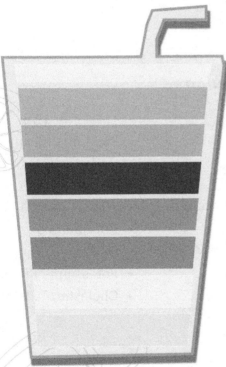

- **1/3 cup cooked oats**
- **1/3 cup raspberries**
- **1 cup spinach**
- **1/3 cup blackberries**
- **1/4 of an avocado**
- **1/3 cup blueberries**
- **1/3 cup probiotic yogurt**
- **8 fl oz Icy Green Tea**

! **Add:** 1 fresh squeezed lemon.

Nutritional :

- Total Fat: 15 g
- Sodium: 86 mg
- Carbohydrates: 56 g
- Dietary fiber: 11,5g
- Total sugars: 21 g
- Protein : 10 g
- Calcium : 36 mg
- Potassium : 762 mg
- Cholesterol : 7 mg

1 cups   **5 mins**   **364 kcal**

*Blend all the ingredients into your blender until smooth.

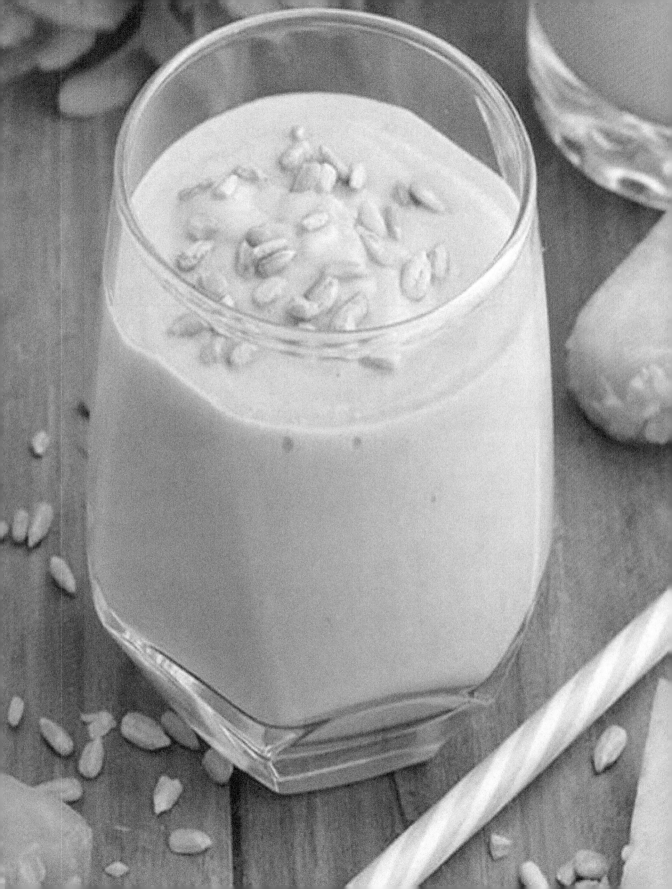

Papaya, Pear and Yoghurt

This smoothie will provide energy to you in a delicious way. You can have this for your breakfast and be energetic the whole day. All the ingredients here give specific color and texture to your smoothie.

Ingredients :

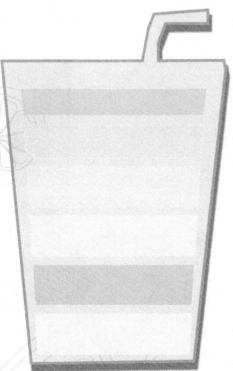

- **1 tablespoon honey**
- **2 tbsp sunflower seeds**
- **1 cup pear cubes**
- **½ cup Greek yogurt**
- **2 cups papaya cubes**
- **½ cup coconut milk**

Nutritional :

- Total Fat: 11,8 g
- Sodium: 22 mg
- Carbohydrates: 23 g
- Dietary fiber: 3,3g
- Total sugars: 0 g
- Protein : 5,1 g
- Calcium : 165 mg
- Potassium : 214 mg
- Cholesterol : 10 mg

! **Add:** 1 fresh squeezed lemon.

3 cups   **10 mins**   **231 kcal**

*Blend all the ingredients into your blender until smooth.

Papaya Mango

This smoothie can be a wholesome breakfast when in a hurry. It will provide all the nutrition and will keep you full of the essence of mango. The antioxidant elements will prevent oxidation in organs, cells, etc.

Ingredients :

- **Crushed ice while serving**
- **1 tablespoon sugar**
- **1 tbsp lemon juice**
- **1 cup papaya puree**
- **1 cup mango pulp**

Nutritional :

- Total Fat: 0,8 g
- Sodium: 40,2 mg
- Carbohydrates: 42 g
- Dietary fiber: 2,5 g
- Total sugars: 0 g
- Protein : 1,9 g
- Calcium : 57,9 mg
- Potassium : 395 mg
- Cholesterol : 0 mg

 2 cups   **7 mins**   **182 kcal**

*Blend them until you get a smooth and creamy texture. Enjoy!

Black Raspberry

You can have this tasty smoothie any time of the day, and it is a healthy antioxidant smoothie. WithThis becomes a must-try when black raspberry is in the base of the curd, honey, and vanilla essence. Tastier and healthier, this combination makes this a must-try recipe.

Ingredients :

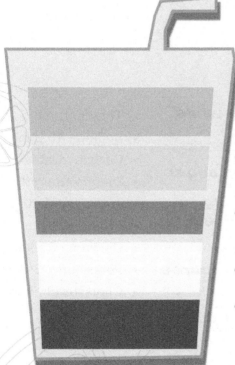

- **½ cup ice-cubes**
- **¾ tablespoon honey**
- **¼ tbsp vanilla essence**
- **½ cup curd**
- **1 cup black raspberry**

Nutritional :

- Total Fat: 3,8 g
- Sodium: 10,6 mg
- Carbohydrates: 18 g
- Dietary fiber: 5,3 g
- Total sugars: 0 g
- Protein : 3,2 g
- Calcium : 126 mg
- Potassium : 173 mg
- Cholesterol : 8 mg

 2 cups   **5 mins**   **124 kcal**

*Blend all the ingredients into your blender until smooth.

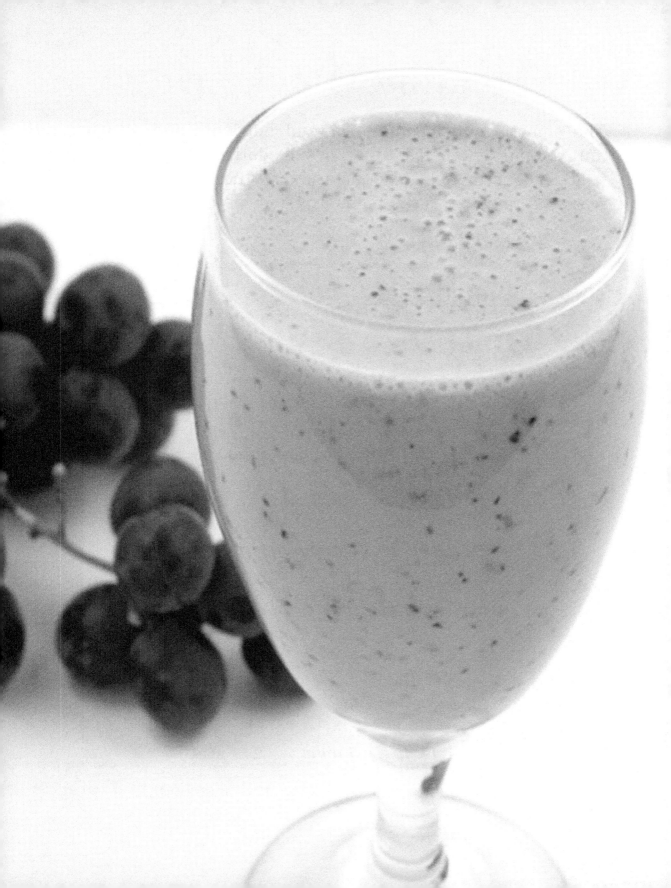

Healthy Black Grape

The smoothie is rich in flavor and nutrients and also has an antioxidant that helps to relieve oxidative stress. Also, black grapes help to keep the arteries of the heart. This mouth-watering smoothie is rich in energy and protein.

Ingredients :

- **½ cup ice-cubes**
- **½ cup curd**
- **½ cup black grapes**
- **½ cup milk**

Nutritional :

- Total Fat: 13 g
- Sodium: 38 mg
- Carbohydrates: 10 g
- Dietary fiber: 0 g
- Total sugars: 0 g
- Protein : 8,6 g
- Calcium : 420 mg
- Potassium : 180 mg
- Cholesterol : 32 mg

 1 cups   **5 mins**   **243 kcal**

*Blend all the ingredients into your blender until smooth.

Apricot Apple Smoothie

The apricot apple smoothie keeps you full of energy the whole day. The ingredients like banana, nuts, apple, and soy milk make a mixture full of nutrition and thus is a perfect way to be energetic.

Ingredients :

- **4 tablespoon curd**
- **4 cups apple juice**
- **4 medium apples**
- **4 medium peaches**
- **18-20 apricots (wet)**
- **4 medium banana**
- **2 cups milk**

Nutritional :

- Total Fat: 3,2 g
- Sodium: 91,7 mg
- Carbohydrates: 64 g
- Dietary fiber: 10 g
- Total sugars: 0 g
- Protein : 3,9 g
- Calcium : 65,7 mg
- Potassium : 388 mg
- Cholesterol : 1,6 mg

 6 cups   **5 mins**   **304 kcal**

*Blend them until you get a smooth and creamy texture. Enjoy!

Green Blueberry Smoothie

It provides you a tangy and luscious texture with blueberries. The wholesome ingredients bring a sweet taste to your mouth, bringing you lots of energy. It reduces cell damage that taken place due to the free radicals.

Ingredients :

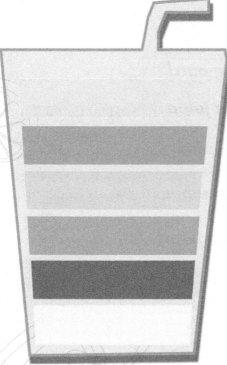

- *1 tbsp honey*
- *¼ tbsp vanilla essence*
- *2 tbsp cooking oats*
- *¾ cup spinach*
- *¾ cup frozen blueberry*
- *¾ cup almond milk*

Nutritional :

- Total Fat: 1,8 g
- Sodium: 34,3 mg
- Carbohydrates: 17 g
- Dietary fiber: 2,9 g
- Total sugars: 0 g
- Protein : 2,2 g
- Calcium : 85,7 mg
- Potassium : 117 mg
- Cholesterol : 0 mg

2 cups **5 mins**   **87 kcal**

*Blend all the ingredients into your blender until smooth.

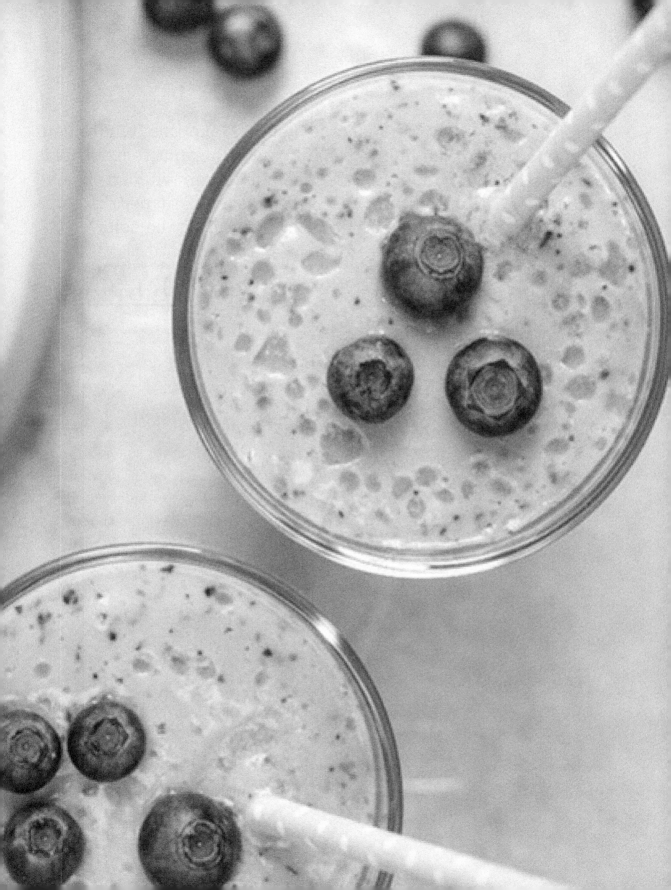

Cranberry-Banana Antioxidant

Don't have enough ingredients at hand? Make this 3-ingredient smoothie that is rich in antioxidants and other nutrients. This is a refreshing smoothie that is super high in vitamin C and potassium. The benefits of this smoothie make it perfect for a post-workout booster. It also helps in fighting off the cold.

Ingredients :

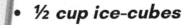

- **½ cup ice-cubes**

- **3/4 cup cranberries**

- **1 large, frozen banana**

- **3/4 cup coconut water**

Nutritional :

- Total Fat: 0,4 g
- Sodium: 1 mg
- Carbohydrates: 34 g
- Dietary fiber: 6,1 g
- Total sugars: 17,4 g
- Protein : 1,3 g
- Calcium : 19 mg
- Potassium : 563 mg
- Cholesterol : 0 mg

 1 cups   **5 mins**   **170 kcal**

*Blend all the ingredients into your blender until smooth.

Dragon Fruit Bowl

This dragon fruit smoothie bowl makes for a perfect snack, breakfast, or dessert. The dragon fruit (or pitaya) bowl is full of antioxidants and is low-calorie and, nutrient-dense. It is one of the best vegan smoothie bowls out there and perfect for dessert. Must try!

Ingredients :

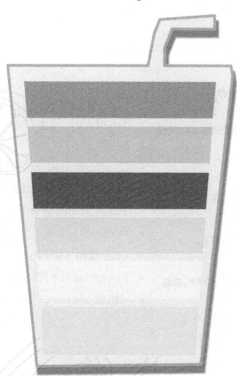

- **Almonds, walnuts**
- **Almond Butter**
- **Dark chocolate chips**
- **Toasted Coconut Granola**
- **Coconut flakes**
- **1 dragon fruit**

Nutritional :

- Total Fat: 14 g
- Sodium: 70 mg
- Carbohydrates: 62 g
- Dietary fiber: 6 g
- Total sugars: 44 g
- Protein : 3 g
- Calcium : 28 mg
- Potassium : 823 mg
- Cholesterol : 0 mg

! **OPTIONAL:** you can replace <u>dragon fruit</u> with kiwi, berries, bananas. <u>Almonds</u> with: hemp or pumpkin seeds.

1 cups   **5 mins**   **375 kcal**

*Blend all the ingredients into your blender until smooth.

Purple Smoothie

This plant-based purple smoothie is a simple recipe featuring purple superfoods like blackberries, acai, grapes, and goji berries. A powerful purple blast of antioxidants! Throw in many seeds, nuts or coconut yogurt, and some healthy fats, and you have got yourself a wholesome meal.

Ingredients :

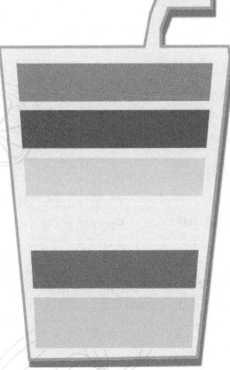

- *1 tsp dried goji*
- *1 packet frozen acai puree*
- *½ cup grapes*
- *1 small banana*
- *½ cup blackberries*
- *1-2 ice cubes*

Nutritional :

- Total Fat: 9 g
- Sodium: 10 mg
- Carbohydrates: 57 g
- Dietary fiber: 11 g
- Total sugars: 30 g
- Protein : 8 g
- Calcium : 28 mg
- Potassium : 823 mg
- Cholesterol : 78 mg

1 cups   **5 mins**   **317 kcal**

*Blend all the ingredients into your blender until smooth.

Chapter 6
Five Basic Daily Exercises

When you are on a journey to lose weight, you have to consider every aspect of it. You will lose weight through healthy eating, but you will also gain it back if you don't take proper care to maintain it. To make sure you get the desired result and maintain it, you need to exercise. Exercise doesn't mean training for hours. Instead, you just need a few minutes out of your day to start, and that would do the trick. Here are five exercises you can do daily to lose weight faster and maintain it, even if you are a beginner.

Before you start doing these exercises, make sure to do some stretching so that your body doesn't become sore. You can do a bunch of stretching exercises like neck and shoulder rolls, wrist circles, arm swings, big arm circles, hip circles, lateral and forward leg swings, and bent-over twists. Do these stretches for 5-10 seconds each before exercising? If an exercise starts to hurt or feel bad, please stop doing it. If you have any special considerations when it comes to exercise, consult your doctor.

STOMACH VACUUM

The stomach vacuum exercise is one of the best exercises to get a slim waistline and abs. This exercise requires you to pull in your internal organs, which improves your core strength and activates your abdominal muscles. You can do this exercise while sitting, standing, or kneeling. Just push all the air out of your lungs and pull in your stomach as much you can. Hold this position for five seconds and repeat the cycle 3-5 times.

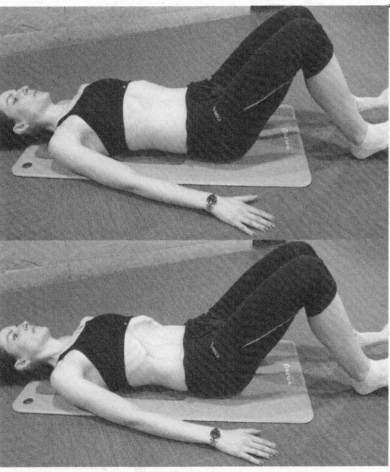

Benefits:

1. Stabilizes your spine and hips.
2. Improves your metabolism.
3. Supports your digestive system.
4. Regulates endocrine system.

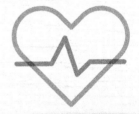

Note: Do not do this exercise if you have hernia, or you have high blood pressure.

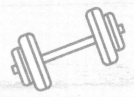

PLANK EXERCISES

Planks work as one of the best core-strengthening exercises. But do you know that planks are beneficial for the whole body? Just a few plank exercises such as elbow planks, straight arm planks, reverse planks, and forearm side planks (left & right) give you enough energy to get through the day. To start, hold each position for 30-60 seconds and move on to the next one.

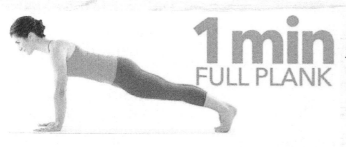

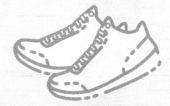

Benefits:

1. Improvement in body balance and posture.
2. Strengthening of core, shoulders, joints, and pelvis.
3. Better body flexibility.
4. Better metabolism.

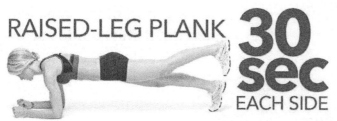

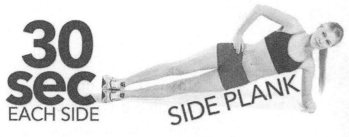

Note: Do not do planks if you have shoulder pain or back problems.

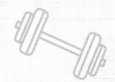

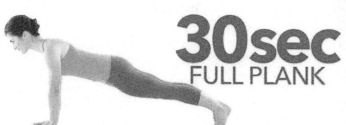

HIGH KNEES

The high knee is an intense exercise that is great for kicking in some daily cardio. Just 20 high knees are enough to improve your stamina, strength, momentum, and flexibility. To do this, be in a standing position and start running in place with your knees as high as possible. Do at least 20 reps and repeat if you want.

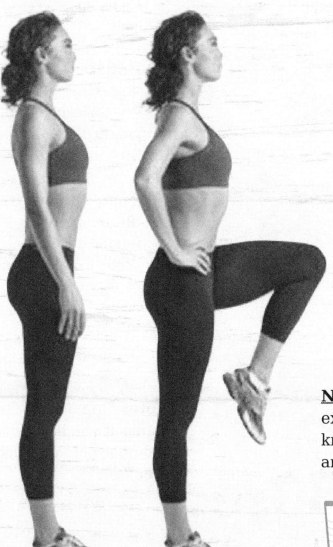

Doing high knees regularly:

1. Strengthens your core.
2. Improves your running technique.
3. Strengthens leg and glute muscles.
4. It Burns a lot of calories.

Note: Don't do this exercise if you have knee pain or knee arthritis.

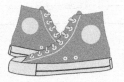

SQUATS

Squats is a powerful exercise that targets your legs, glutes, core, and lower back muscles. You can do squats in different ways, each of which has different benefits. However, to do the traditional squats, all you have to do is stand with your knees slightly bent to push your hips backward. Make sure your back is straight. Now straighten out your arms in front and try to reach a 90-degree angle, just like how you sit on a chair. Once you reach the position, move back up. Do this 25-30 times every day to see the results.

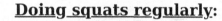

Doing squats regularly:
   1. Strengthens the calves, legs, and glutes.
   2. Strengthens your knees and back.
   3. Burns fat.
   4. Improves flexibility.

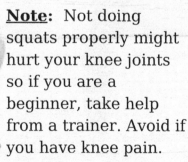

Note: Not doing squats properly might hurt your knee joints so if you are a beginner, take help from a trainer. Avoid if you have knee pain.

TIP-TOE SQUIRTS

Tiptoe squirts are very beneficial for the lower body. The pressure you put on your toes and calves during this exercise engages your core and improves your posture. To do this, stand up with your feet slightly apart. Bend a little lower into a squat, and then lift your heels. Now, stand back up and repeat the cycle. Do at least 10 reps.

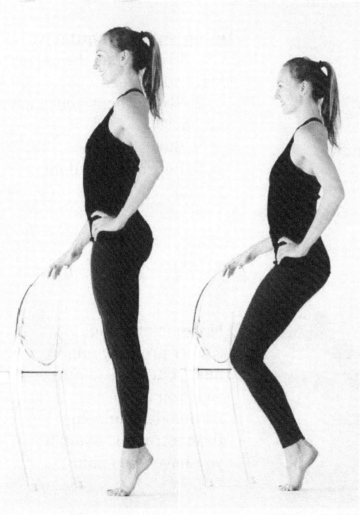

Benefits:
1. Improves your foot health.
2. Improves balance and posture.
3. Helps to relieve ankle pains and stress fractures.
4. Strengthens your inner thighs.

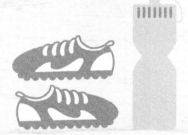

Note: If you have knee issues, consult with your doctor before doing this exercise.

Start Seeing Results in Just Five Days

Hey, you made it! You have reached the final segment of this book. Now, what's left is to apply all that you have read and make it into a daily routine. It's tough, I know. I had the same issues when I was starting. But, as soon as I developed a routine, things became easier. Developing a routine is the way to achieve your goals and maintain your achieved target in the long term. To get results faster and to strengthen the results, I strongly recommend that you combine the smoothie diet with daily exercise. Following a good diet with regular exercise can get you results in just five days. I will guide you in the smallest details through your first five days in the 5 days kick-start plan right after this chapter. And, with the methods and recipes given in this book, it is a guarantee that you will see results. However, to achieve the desired results, I strongly suggest that you follow this 5-day diet and exercise routine at least four times in a row. In 20 days, you will be able to see a nice difference in yourself, not just from the outside but from the inside as well. They say that you can make or break a habit in 21 days – and what an essential habit it is. The best part is that it is easy and you can even repeat this practice whenever you want.

The biggest improvement you will see is with your discipline. You will become focused, habitual in your efforts, and mindful of your body and will take care of it without even realizing it. The best part about a smoothie diet is that you can incorporate it into any meal. However, most people get skeptical about whether they should have smoothies before or after a workout. Well, both have their fair share of benefits. Having a pre-workout smoothie 1-3 hours before your workout will provide you the fuel you need for your body to perform at its best. Post-workout smoothies, on the other hand, are more complex. Its role is to replenish and rejuvenate your body from the workout. You can have a post-workout smoothie 30-60 mins after your workout to give your body the energy to recover. So, if you plan on doing an intense workout session, fuel your body up with a nourishing pre-workout smoothie.

Any kind of smoothie, in general, is much better than a slice of pizza or that scoop of vanilla ice cream.

Just switch your junk cravings with smoothies, and soon, you will not even think about having ice cream for a snack. This book has everything to help you get started and stay right on track. Here are some of the benefits you will obtain if you follow the instructions given in this book and following the 5-day routine I'm proposing in the next chapter :

● Lose weight up to five pounds: With the right diet and exercise mentioned in this book, you can lose up to five pounds in just five days. Just weigh yourself at the beginning and the end of this program and see the difference for yourself!

●Lose up to one inch: With this program, you can shred up to one inch off your waist to get a slimmer waistline.

●Better sleep: Switching to a healthier diet and exercising takes a lot of stress away, resulting in better sleep. Record your sleep cycles for five days and notice the improvement. You will be amazed to see how better your sleep cycle becomes.

●Blood pressure control: An increase in blood pressure often happens due to consuming unhealthy foods, full of added sugars, carbs, and chemicals. Therefore, switching to a healthy diet keeps all the toxicity and inflammation away from your body and keeps your blood pressure under control.

● Improves your mood: The chemicals present in unhealthy foods disturb your mood in a lot of ways. But, by following a healthy routine like the one mentioned in the book, you will feel much better both physically and mentally in just five days.

It is hard to believe that just five days of diet along with five days of exercise can transform your body in the ways mentioned above. If you think the same, try the plan yourself and see the results. It is just five days, so it will not take much time off your schedule. You will only believe it if you try!

Quick disclaimer: The sole purpose of this book is to help you start your fitness journey off on the right foot and achieve desired results.

However, if you don't follow the instructions diligently, you are not going to get the results you want. Your transformation depends on your dedication and how badly you want to become a better version of yourself. So, apart from following the diet and exercise plans mentioned in the book, you also need to take care of some other things yourself. These include:

- Staying away from fast foods means no pizza, burger, fries, or your favorite dessert.
- No alcohol. Alcohol works as a roadblock and can revert all your efforts right away.
- No drugs, even when you are not trying to lose weight.
- Avoiding store-bought "health" food—they do no good.

Avoiding all of the things mentioned will not only help you lose that extra fat but will also support your wellbeing. This is not a short-term change we are talking about, this is a change in your lifestyle. A lifestyle change can help you stay fit and healthy for the rest of your life. All you have to do is stick to your routine. Even if you get demotivated sometimes, remind yourself why you started in the first place and get back on track. The journey is surely not easy, but the results make it worth the effort. So, what are you waiting for? Get started on this new chapter in your life and see how it goes. I promise it will be much better than you think!

Diet Plan for 5 Days.

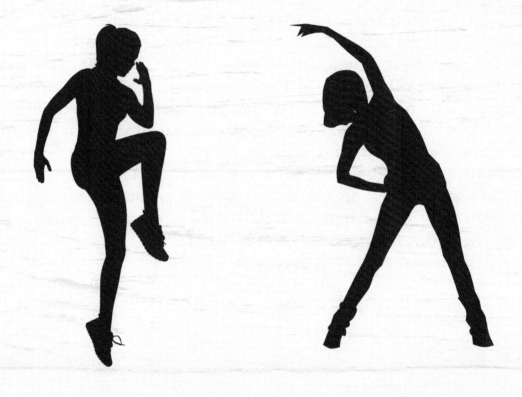

BODY MEASUREMENTS

BEFORE

DATE _____

NECK _____

CHEST _____

LEFT ARM _____

RIGHT ARM _____

WAIST _____

HIPS _____

LEFT THIGH _____

RIGHT THIGH _____

LEFT CALF _____

RIGHT CALF _____

WEIGHT _____

AFTER

DATE _____

NECK _____

CHEST _____

LEFT ARM _____

RIGHT ARM _____

WAIST _____

HIPS _____

LEFT THIGH _____

RIGHT THIGH _____

LEFT CALF _____

RIGHT CALF _____

WEIGHT _____

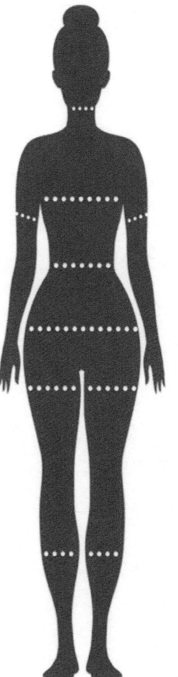

BEFORE   AFTER

DATE_____   DATE_____

NECK_____   NECK_____

CHEST_____   CHEST_____

LEFT ARM_____   LEFT ARM_____

RIGHT ARM_____   RIGHT ARM_____

WAIST_____   WAIST_____

HIPS_____   HIPS_____

LEFT THIGH_____   LEFT THIGH_____

RIGHT THIGH_____   RIGHT THIGH_____

LEFT CALF_____   LEFT CALF_____

RIGHT CALF_____   RIGHT CALF_____

WEIGHT_____   WEIGHT_____

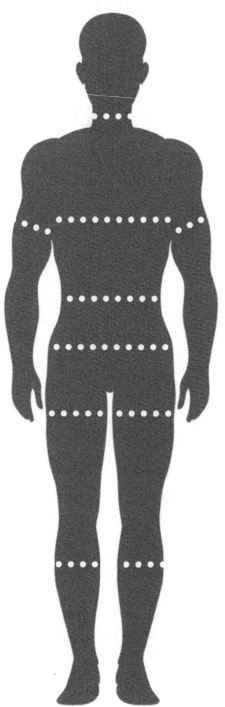

DATE *FIRST DAY*

M T W T F

H₂O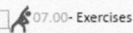

TODAY'S SCHEDULE

- ❏ A cup of warm water after waking up
  06.00-06.30
- ❏ 07.00- Exercises
  - ❏ Stretching
  - ❏ Vaccum
- ❏ 07.30-08.00 -Smoothie
  Papaya, Pear&Yoghurt
- ❏ Breakfast *2 boiled eggs+porridge+1*
  08.30-9.00 *cucumber+tea/coffee*
- ❏ Snack 1 *fruits by 12.00+ water*
  10.00-11.00
- ❏ Lunch *sckinless chichen+ripe*
  13.00-14.00 *vegetable+water*
- ❏ Snack 2 *2-3 dried plums+ tea/coffee*
  16.00-17.00
- ❏ 17.30 –Exercises
  - ❏ Planking
  - ❏ High Knee
  - ❏ Squats
  - ❏ Tip Toe Squirts
- ❏ 18.00-18.30 Smoothie
  Papaya& Mango
- ❏ Dinner *baking fish+salat+water*
  19.00-20.00

SHOPPING LIST

SMOOTHIES:

Papaya- 3 p.
Mango- 1 p.
Lemon- 1 p.
Pear- 2 p.
Yogurt- 150gr
Coconut milk- 150 ml
Sunflowers seeds- 100 gr

MEAL:

Egg- 2p.
Cucumber-1p.
Porridge-1pack
Chicken-200 gr.
Fish-300 gr
Dried plums- 2/3p.
Salat-1/2 of dish
Vegetable-1/2 of dish
Fruits-2p.(excluded- banana,grapes)

MY DAILY CHECK-IN

| My Mood | ❏ ❏ | Heart beat | [   ] |
| Sleep well ? | ❏ ❏ | Blood pressure | [   ] |

DATE *SECOND DAY*

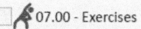

TODAY'S SCHEDULE

- ❑ A cup of warm water after waking up
  06.00-06.30

- ❑ 🏃 07.00 - Exercises

  - ❑ Stretching
  - ❑ Vaccum

- ❑ 07.30-08.00 Smoothie
  Vitamin C Antioxidanta

- ❑ Breakfast *2 toast with a cream cheese*
  08.30-9.00   *1 cucumber+tea/coffee*
- ❑ Snack 1   *fruits by 12.00+ water*
  10.00-11.00
- ❑ Lunch   *baking chicken legs+baking*
  13.00-14.00   *cabbage+ water*
- ❑ Snack 2   *handful of nuts+ tea/coffee*
  16.00-17.00

- ❑ 🏃 17.30 –Exercises

  - ❑ Planking
  - ❑ High Knee
  - ❑ Squats
  - ❑ Tip Toe Squirts

- ❑ 18.00-18.30 Smoothie
  Black Raspberry

- ❑ Dinner   *sckinless chicken +salat*
  19.00-20.00   *+water*

H₂O ⬡⬡⬡⬡⬡⬡⬡

SHOPPING LIST

SMOOTHIES:

Apple- 1 p.
Raspberry-200 gr
Avocado- 1 p.
Beet-1small
Lemon- 1 p.
Celery- 1 stick
Curd- 150gr
Almond milk- 150 ml
Strawberries- 200 gr

MEAL:

Toast- 2p.
Cucumber-1p.
Cream cheese-100gr
Chicken leg-1p.
Sckinless chicken-200 gr
Cabbage- 200 gr
Salat-1/2 of dish
Nuts-100gr
Fruits-2p.(excluded- banana, grapes)

MY DAILY CHECK-IN

My Mood ❑ ❑ ❑ ☹   Heart beat ▭

Sleep well ? ❑ ❑ ❑ ☹   Blood pressure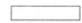

DATE *THIRD DAY*
M T W T F

H2O ◌ ◌ ◌ ◌ ◌ ◌ ◌

TODAY'S SCHEDULE

❑ A cup of warm water after waking up
06.00-06.30

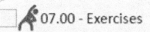 07.00 - Exercises

❑ Stretching
❑ Vaccum

07.30-08.00 Smoothie
Antioxidant Triple-Berry

❑ Breakfast *1 banana+ yogurt +oatmeal*
08.30-9.00   *1 cucumber+tea/coffee*
❑ Snack 1 *handful of nuts+ water*
10.00-11.00
❑ Lunch *baking chicken legs +*
13.00-14.00   *green salat+ water*
❑ Snack 2 *2/3 dried plums+ tea/coffee*
16.00-17.00

17.30 – Exercises

❑ Planking
❑ High Knee
❑ Squats
❑ Tip Toe Squirts

18.00-18.30 Smoothie
Blueberry Ginger Detox

❑ Dinner *cream of chicken broth*
19.00-20.00   *+2 toast*

SHOPPING LIST

SMOOTHIES:
Banana- 1 p.
Blackberries- 150 gr
Raspberry-150 gr
Blueberries- 200gr
Spinach- 300 gr
Yogurt- 150gr
Almond milk- 250 ml
Almond butter-1tbsp
Hempseeds&Flaxseeds-1tbsp
Ginger juice- 3 tbsp

MEAL:
Toast- 2p.
Cucumber-1p.
Banana-1p.
Yogurt-150 gr.
Oatmeal-150 gr.
Chicken leg-1p.
Sckinless chicken-200 gr
Dried plums- 2/3 p.
Green salat-1/2 of dish
Nuts-100gr
Fruits-2p.(excluded- grapes)

MY DAILY CHECK-IN

My Mood ❑ ☺ ❑ 😐 ❑ ☹   Heart beat [   ]

Sleep well ? ❑ ☺ ❑ 😐 ❑ ☹   Blood pressure [   ]

DATE *FOURTH DAY*

M T W T F

TODAY'S SCHEDULE

- ☐ A cup of warm water after waking up
  06.00-06.30

☐ 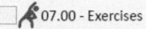 **07.00 - Exercises**

- ☐ Stretching
- ☐ Vaccum

☐ 07.30-08.00 Smoothie
Silky Skin

- ☐ Breakfast 2 toast+cream chees+ 2 eggs
  08.30-9.00   1 cucumber+tea/coffee
- ☐ Snack 1   fruits by 12.00+ water
  10.00-11.00
- ☐ Lunch   skinless chichen + baking
  13.00-14.00   vegetable+ water
- ☐ Snack 2   handful of nuts+ tea/coffee
  16.00-17.00

☐ 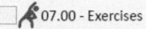 **17.30 – Exercises**

- ☐ Planking
- ☐ High Knee
- ☐ Squats
- ☐ Tip Toe Squirts

☐ 18.00-18.30 Smoothie
Vegan Detox& Fat Burn

- ☐ Dinner   baking fish+ baking
  19.00-20.00   cabbage

SHOPPING LIST

H₂O ⬡⬡⬡⬡⬡⬡⬡⬡

SMOOTHIES:
Carrot- 2 bigs.
Apricot- 1p.
Dried apricots-100 gr
Cinnamon- ½ tsp
Honey- 1 tbsp.
Yogurt- 150gr
Tomato-1p.
Celery-1 stik
Coriander leaves-handful
Lemon- 1 p.
Pepper-1 tsp
Cumin seed powder- 1 tsp
MEAL:
Toast- 2p.
Cucumber-1p.
Eggs- 2p.
Cream cheese-150 gr.
Fish-300gr.
Sckinless chicken-200 gr
Nuts- 100 gr.
Vegetable-1/2 of dish
Cabbage 200 gr.
Fruits-2p.(excluded- grapes)

MY DAILY CHECK-IN

My Mood   ☐ 😊 ☐ 😐 ☐ 🙁   Heart beat   [   ]

Sleep well ? ☐ 😊 ☐ 😐 ☐ 🙁   Blood pressure [   ]

DATE *FIFTH DAY*

M T W T F

H₂O ⬡⬡⬡⬡⬡⬡⬡⬡

TODAY'S SCHEDULE

- ☐ A cup of warm water after waking up
  06.00-06.30

☐ 🏃 **07.00 - Exercises**

- ☐ Stretching
- ☐ Vaccum

☐ **07.30-08.00 Smoothie**
Tropical Green

- ☐ Breakfast *1 yogurt+ 2 eggs*
  08.30-9.00 *1 cucumber+tea/coffee*
- ☐ Snack 1 *fruits by 12.00+ water*
  10.00-11.00
- ☐ Lunch *turkey or chicken soup +*
  13.00-14.00 *2 toast+chilly+ water*
- ☐ Snack 2 *2-3 dried plums + tea/coffee*
  16.00-17.00

☐ 🏃 **17.30 – Afternoon Exercises**

- ☐ Planking
- ☐ High Knee
- ☐ Squats
- ☐ Tip Toe Squirts

☐ **18.00-18.30 Smoothie**
Beet Detox

- ☐ Dinner *baking chicken leg+ mix salat*
  19.00-20.00 *+wather*

SHOPPING LIST

SMOOTHIES:

Beet- 1 small.
Banana- 2 p.
Blueberries-100 gr
Strawberries- 300 gr
Mango- 1 p.
Orange- 1 big
Coconut milk-150 ml
Matcha powder-2 tbsp

MEAL:

Yogurt- 150 gr.
Cucumber-1p.
Eggs- 2p.
Turkey/Chicken-200 gr.
Toast-2 p.
Chilly-1 p.
Chicken leg-1 p.
Dried plums- 2/3 p.
Mix salat-1/2 of dish
Fruits-2p.(excluded- grapes)

MY DAILY CHECK-IN

My Mood ☐   ☐   ☐   Heart beat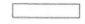

Sleep well ? ☐   ☐   ☐   Blood pressure ▭

MY WEEKLY REFLECTION

My Mood ☐ 😊 ☐ 😐 ☐ 😕   Heart beat [＿＿＿]

Sleep well ? ☐ 😊 ☐ 😐 ☐ 😕   Blood pressure [＿＿＿]

I was successful in

_____

_____

_____

_____

_____

I had an inssue with

_____

_____

_____

_____

_____

My goal next week is to...

_____

_____

_____

_____

YOU GOT THIS !!!

Conclusion

Here we are, at the end of this book and the journey you started with me, even though this is not nearly the end of your journey. At first, this book was not meant to be a detailed version of everything you need to know before starting your fitness journey. It was going to be a simple smoothie recipe book. But that made me think "how is this going to be any different from all the other recipe books out there?" People don't just need to know what they have to eat to lose weight, but they should also know why they have to eat it. Through this book, I have tried to answer the 'why' in the best way possible. Everything in this book, whether it is the ingredients of the smoothie, benefits of each ingredient, nutrient content in each ingredient, or wholesome smoothie recipes, is carefully curated to make sure that you understand what you put in your body and how it is going to affect your physical and mental wellbeing.

People often think that smoothies are all about fruits, and they excite your sugar levels. But that's not true. A smoothie is a mixture of all types of ingredients—fruits, vegetables, and whole foods. That's why we have included all kinds of smoothies in this book to show you its versatile nature. You can even make all-vegetable smoothies if you want, like the ones mentioned in the book. The idea is to incorporate the required amounts of nutrients through a simple and quick process, and nothing is better than smoothies for that.

I also included some beneficial exercises for you to do along with your diet. The exercises are simple yet effective. They target specific areas of your body and help improve your strength. Doing these exercises daily will accelerate weight loss and help you maintain your achieved target. The diet program and exercises in this book aim to help everyone, whether they are just starting or want a little quick-fix to get back on their healthy schedule. If you follow the 5 days program, you will start to see results yourself. Of course, you will not magically transform into a different person, but you will start to notice some change. Give yourself some time to see the magic happening, though you will feel better quickly. It is all about being consistent and disciplined. Just a few days of determination can change your mood and your body, and soon, it will become a habit. Your cravings will decrease, your heart will be healthy, and your mind will be at peace. Isn't that what we all want?

It is your turn now. It is up to you to continue this journey now, especially when your motivation level is at its peak. So, if you are feeling motivated enough, welcome this new phase in your life—one that will hopefully stay with you for the long term. All the best!

Get our new release for FREE!

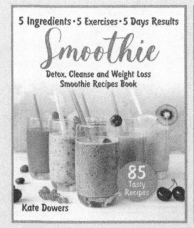 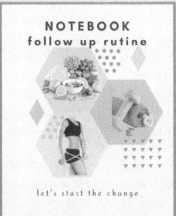 

Sing up to our newsletter to get the future release absolutely Free!

https://mailchi.mp/b7abe36ee0fc/kate-dowers

References

- Arnarson, A. (2019 7). Antioxidants Explained in Simple Terms. Healthline. https://www.healthline.com/nutrition/antioxidants-explained#free-radicals

- Biswas, C. (2016, September 30). Top 25 Detox Smoothies For Weight Loss. STYLECRAZE. https://www.stylecraze.com/articles/top-detox-smoothie-recipes/#MetabolismBoosterGreenSmoothie

- Bryan, L. (2020, December 29). 20+ Best Smoothie Recipes. Downshiftology. https://downshiftology.com/best-smoothie-recipes/

- DocOnline. (2019, February 3). What is Detox, and How do you know if your body needs it? PART 1. Www.doconline.com. https://www.doconline.com/blog/what-is-detox-and-how-do-you-know-if-your-body-needs-it

- Fellizar, K. (2018, October 17). 7 Subtle Signs Of Toxin Overload In Your Body. Bustle. https://www.bustle.com/p/7-subtle-signs-of-toxin-overload-in-your-body-12137633

- Funke, L. (2020, April 1). 100+ Healthy Smoothie Recipes. Fit Foodie Finds. https://fitfoodiefinds.com/100-healthy-smoothie-recipes/

- Getmymettle. (2020, December 28). Stomach Vacuum Exercise [Complete Guide]. Getmymettle. https://getmymettle.com/stomach-vacuum/stomach-vacuum/

- Healthline. (2021, January 7). The 5 Best Blenders for Smoothies. Healthline. https://www.healthline.com/nutrition/best-blender-for-smoothies#our-picks

- Heathers, J. (2019, May 4). 5 significant reasons to lose weight. (Why isn't the media covering these?). Precision Nutrition; Precision Nutrition. https://www.precisionnutrition.com/reasons-to-lose-weight

- Heathessentials. (2021, February 12). How to Make Healthy and Delicious Smoothies. Health Essentials from Cleveland Clinic.

https://health.clevelandclinic.org/how-to-make-healthy-and-delicious-
smoothies/

- https://www.facebook.com/asweetpeachef. (2020, March 25). 5 High Protein Fruit Smoothies for Weight Loss (5 Ingredients or Less). A Sweet Pea Chef. https://www.asweetpeachef.com/high-protein-fruit-smoothie-recipes/
- Jane, M. (2017, June 15). Fresh vs. Frozen Fruit and Vegetables — Which Are Healthier? Healthline; Health line Media. https://www.healthline.com/nutrition/fresh-vs-frozen-fruit-and-vegetables
- Jones, A. (2016, September 19). 8 Detox Smoothie Recipes for a Fast Weight Loss | Lose Weight. Lose Weight by Eating. https://loseweightbyeating.com/detox-smoothie-recipes-weight-loss-cleanse/
- Leal, D. (2021, March 3). 5-Minute Daily Plank Workout. Verywell Fit. https://www.verywellfit.com/five-minute-daily-plank-workout-4588742
- Lindberg, S. (2019, September 11). Benefits of Squats, Variations, and Muscles Worked. Healthline. https://www.healthline.com/health/exercise-fitness/squats-benefits#overhead-squats
- Lobo, V., Patil, A., Phatak, A., & Chandra, N. (2010). Free radicals, antioxidants, and functional foods: Impact on human health. Pharmacognosy Reviews, 4(8), 118. https://doi.org/10.4103/0973-7847.70902
- MacMillan, A. (2015, February 12). How Your Taste Buds Can Help You Lose Weight? Health.com. https://www.health.com/weight-loss/how-your-taste-buds-can-help-you-lose-weight
- Milliner-Waddell, M. B., Hilary Reid, Jenna. (2021, February 22). The Best Blenders for Smoothies, According to Chefs and Smoothie Fanatics. The Strategist. https://nymag.com/strategist/article/best-blender-for-smoothies.html

- N., J. (2021, January 25). 25 Detox Smoothies to Cleanse Your Body. Swanson Health Hub. https://swanson-blog-preview.groupby.cloud/blog/detox-smoothie-cleanse/
- October 8, S. L., & 2020. (2020, October 8). 11 Tricks for the Best-Ever Smoothie. Eat This Not That. https://www.eatthis.com/best-smoothie-tips/
- Padda, I. (2020, December 3). 10 Warning Signs of Toxic Overload in the Body. EMediHealth. https://www.emedihealth.com/toxic-overload-warning-signs.html
- Pinterest. (2018). 19 Best Antioxidant Smoothie ideas | smoothie drinks, healthy smoothies, smoothies. Pinterest. https://in.pinterest.com/shuber99/antioxidant-smoothie/
- Pro Cheer Life. (2016). High Knees Exercise: Benefits and Variations. PRO CHEER LIFE. https://procheerlife.mykajabi.com/blog/high-knees-exercise-benefits-and-variations
- Raman, R. (2018, March 12). 12 Healthy Foods High in Antioxidants. Healthline. https://www.healthline.com/nutrition/foods-high-in-antioxidants#TOC_TITLE_HDR_2
- September 23, O. T., & 2017. (2017, September 23). The BEST Smoothies For Weight Loss. Eat This Not That. https://www.eatthis.com/10-smoothie-recipes-weight-loss/
- Tarantino, O. (2016, July 30). 33 Reasons To Lose Weight Besides Fitting Into Your Old Jeans. Eat This Not That; Eat This Not That. https://www.eatthis.com/reasons-to-lose-weight/
- Ware, M. (2018, May 29). Antioxidants: Health benefits and nutritional information. Www.medicalnewstoday.com. https://www.medicalnewstoday.com/articles/301506#benefits
- Winchester Hospital. (n.d.). True or False: Fresh Food Is Better Than Frozen or Canned Food | Winchester Hospital. Www.winchesterhospital.org. https://www.winchesterhospital.org/health-library/article?id=160561

Made in the USA
Monee, IL
17 July 2022

99882757R10096